Atlas of Veterinary Surgical Pathology

Atlas of Veterinary Surgical Pathology

Edited by

Joseph S. Haynes DVM, PhD, DACVP
Professor, Iowa State University, Department of Veterinary Pathology, Ames, IA, USA

WILEY Blackwell

Registered Office

John Wiley & Sons, Inc., 111 River Street, Hoboken, NJ 07030, USA

For details of our global editorial offices, customer services, and more information about Wiley products visit us at www.wiley.com.

Wiley also publishes its books in a variety of electronic formats and by print-on-demand. Some content that appears in standard print versions of this book may not be available in other formats.

Library of Congress Cataloging-in-Publication Data is applied for

Hardback ISBN: 9781119261223

Cover image: Courtesy of Joseph S. Haynes

Cover design by Wiley

Set in 9.5/12.5pt STIXTwoText by Straive, Pondicherry, India

Printed in Singapore

M066033_141222

Contents

List of Contributors

Joseph S. Haynes
Department of Veterinary Pathology, Iowa State University, Ames, IA, USA

Michael J. Yaeger
Department of Veterinary Pathology, Iowa State University, Ames, IA, USA

Preface

This book is intended to be a handy, next-to-the-microscope resource that is a collection of descriptions and comments along with high-quality photomicrographs of lesions that are commonly encountered in our veterinary surgical pathology practice. In this volume, we have focused on lesions in five organ systems: the eye and periocular tissues, bones and joints, the integument, the male reproductive system, and the female reproductive system. In addition, each chapter has a list of references and suggested reading that will supply more detailed information.

Acknowledgments

We would like to acknowledge and thank the many mentors who have helped us to become veterinary pathologists, especially those that are skilled in veterinary surgical pathology. Also, we would like to acknowledge the excellent work of the histotechnologists in the Iowa State University Department of Veterinary Pathology who produced the microscopic sections utilized for the photomicrographs in this book. Finally, we would like to acknowledge our colleagues in the department and elsewhere, with whom we interact and discuss cases – they have made us better veterinary pathologists.

1

Pathology of the Eye and Periocular Tissues

Joseph S. Haynes

Department of Veterinary Pathology, Iowa State University, Ames, IA, USA

Introduction

Surgical pathology of the eye is unique in that the eye is a polarized organ with multiple segments, any of which may develop primary disease. A primary disease in one segment frequently will cause secondary disease in another segment. Microscopic examination of a diseased eye is somewhat analogous to performing a necropsy, in that each segment must be examined independently for lesions similar to the way each organ must be examined in an animal at necropsy, before a final diagnosis can be made.

Prefixation Preparation

In general, eyes removed at surgery and submitted for examination of ocular disease should have the periocular tissues, eyelids, and extraocular muscles removed prior to fixation. This should reveal the sclera and the long posterior ciliary arteries, which extend circumferentially around the globe from the optic nerve; these vessels denote the junction of the dorsal (tapetal) and ventral (nontapetal) portions of the fundus. This is important for the purpose of orienting the globe for sectioning, so that both tapetal and nontapetal fundus can be included in the microscopic slide. If the eye has been removed because of a lesion that involves the periocular or palpebral tissue and evaluation for surgical clearance is warranted, then the globe should not be stripped of periocular tissue, but the specimen should be left intact and the surgical margins should be marked with dye prior to fixation.

Fixation of Eyes for Histopathology

After eyes are removed and prepared, they should be immersed in 10–20× volumes of fixative as quickly as possible. Even a delay of few minutes will result in autolysis, especially of the retina. Several fixatives can be used with good results; however, all have some limitations. Traditionally, eyes were fixed in Bouin's fixative, which provided very good preservation of the globe and all internal segments, and it hardened the globe and thus retained the globe's prefixation turgor and shape. However, because of its environmental hazard, it is no longer routinely used. Davidson's fixative, which is composed of ethanol, formalin, and glacial acetic acid, has replaced Bouin's in our laboratory, and it provides the same level of fixation but much less hazardous than Bouin's. Ten percent neutral buffered formalin (10% NBF), which is the standard fixative for all biopsy and necropsy tissue specimens, can also be used. It is inexpensive; provides good fixation for the cornea, external ocular structures, and the anterior uvea and is not as hazardous as Bouin's fixative. However, it is slow to penetrate the globe, which results in a substantial amount of autolysis in the retina. In addition, it does not preserve the prefixation turgor of the globe; therefore, the globe will partially collapse and be more difficult to accurately section. This lack of rapid globe penetration and loss of turgor can be somewhat overcome by injecting 0.25–0.5 ml of formalin into the vitreous chamber with a 25-gauge needle.

Sectioning

Once the eye is fixed and rinsed, it needs to be sectioned. The globe is oriented so that the cornea is on the cutting board surface and the optic nerve is pointing to the ceiling. With a new razor blade (we use a new disposable microtome blade), the first cut is made lateral to the optic nerve, transecting the long posterior ciliary artery. The cut is continued all the way through the lens and cornea onto the cutting board; when the lens is encountered, the blade is pushed vertically through the lens to help avoid displacing it. Then a second cut is made parallel to the first cut on the medial side of the optic nerve, trying to avoid hitting the lens the second time. This produces a section out of the center of the globe that includes the optic nerve head, lens, tapetal, and nontapetal fundus. This section, along with the lateral and medial calottes (cup-shaped lateral and medial pieces of the globe), should be examined for lesions, such as hemorrhage, exudate, lens luxation, detached retina, and masses. An additional section is cut from the center of each calotte; these are perpendicular to the first section and allow evaluation of all four quadrants of the globe. These sections are placed in appropriately sized cassettes for processing and embedding in paraffin.

Processing and Staining

Once the tissues are processed and embedded, they are sectioned on the microtome to produce sections 3–5 μm thick. These are mounted on glass slides, deparafinized, and stained. **Hematoxylin and eosin (HE)** are the standard stains used for microscopic evaluation. Additional stains that may be helpful to identify certain structures or agents include **PAS stain** (basement membranes, fungi, yeasts, plant material); **GMS stain** (fungi, yeasts), and **Gram's stain** (bacteria). **Immunohistochemistry** is very useful for identifying certain molecules and the cells that contain them. Examples include IHC for coronavirus to confirm Feline infectious peritonitis, or glial fibrillary acidic protein (GFAP) to identify astrocytes in the retina and optic nerve.

Ocular Structure and Development

The eye is a complex structure in the shape of a globe that is designed to take in light from the outside and focus it, so it can be transmitted to the brain and form a visual picture of the world. The main components of the eye are **cornea, uvea (iris, ciliary body, and choroid), lens, retina, sclera,** and **optic nerve** (Figure 1.1). In addition, there are three chambers that are either filled with fluid, called **aqueous humor** (anterior and posterior chamber), or a gelatinous mass of **vitreous body** (vitreous chamber). In addition, the globe is surrounded by a set of periocular tissues that include the **conjunctiva** (bulbar and palpebral), **eyelids, third eyelid, lacrimal glands** and ducts, and **extraocular muscles.** Aqueous humor is produced by the nonpigmented epithelium on the ciliary processes and passes from the posterior chamber through the pupil into the anterior chamber, into the **ciliary cleft,** and ultimately is resorbed by the scleral veins. The **trabecular meshwork** is the complex of channels that forms the walls of the ciliary cleft. The angle formed by the junction of the cornea and iris is the **iridocorneal angle.** In most domestic mammals, the IC angle is spanned by a variably perforated structure, the **pectinate ligament** that originates at the termination of **Descemet's membrane** and inserts on the peripheral

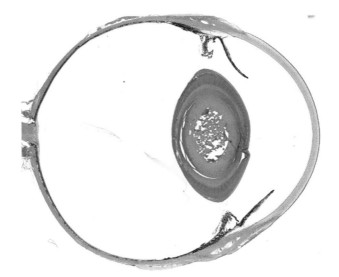

Figure 1.1   Normal canine eye.

aspect of the **iris**. The **lens** is situated behind the iris and is held in place by **zonular fibers** from the **ciliary body**. The **vitreous body** sits behind the lens and fills the vitreous chamber, keeping the **retina** in place. In the vascular tunic of the globe, the **choroid** is the layer external to the retina, and the **sclera** is the densely fibrous external tunic of the globe.

Photons of light enter through the cornea, passing through the stratified squamous epithelium, corneal stroma, and corneal endothelium (inner lining of the cornea). Light continues through the aqueous humor in the anterior and posterior chambers and is then focused by the lens onto the retina. For light to get to the retina, it must pass through the vitreous body (humor). The fluid components of the eye (aqueous and vitreous humors) are important for nutrition and to help maintain the proper shape of the globe and organization of the internal segments; they must remain clear in order to transmit light. Light passes through the inner segment of the retina and is received by the photoreceptors in the outer segment. The photoreceptors (rods and cones) transduce photons of light energy into impulses of electrical energy that are transmitted to the neurons in the inner segment of the retina, especially the ganglion cells. These neurons, in turn, relay impulses through the optic tracts to the vision center in the cerebral cortex, where the visual image is formed.

The eye is formed in a series of steps initiated by an outgrowth of neural tissue from the primitive forebrain; this is the **optic vesicle**. As the optic vesicle grows toward the surface of the embryo, it stimulates the ectoderm to focally thicken into the **lens placode**. The lens placode then enlarges and grows to meet the optic vesicle; as it does this, it will form the **lens vesicle**. The lens vesicle will ultimately give rise to the lens. As the lens vesicle interacts with the optic vesicle, the optic vesicle caves in on itself to form the **optic cup**; this will give rise to the **retina** and **retinal pigment epithelium (RPE)**. This entire group of structures is surrounded by periocular mesenchyme, which will be induced to form the corneal stoma and endothelium, the stroma of the uvea, the sclera, and a transient set of blood vessels that will nourish the developing lens and retina. The development of the periocular mesenchyme into the aforementioned structures depends on appropriate RPE development; if this does not occur, then various ocular anomalies will occur. Such anomalies include **cystic eye**, in which the eye does not develop past the optic vesicle stage, and **microphthalmia**, in which abnormal development produces a small eye with discernible uvea and neuroepithelium that is dysplastic and disorganized (Figure 1.2a, b). There is a wide range in eye size and level of development with microphthalmia. In addition, an eye that is fairly normal in size may have a variety of incompletely developed or dysplastic interior segments, such as goniodysgenesis, choroid hypoplasia, retinal dysplasia, and/or nonattachment; these are frequently lumped together as **multiple ocular defects** (Figure 1.3).

Cornea

The cornea is the most rostral portion of the globe; the junction between the cornea and the sclera is the **limbus**. The cornea is derived from ectoderm and therefore is essentially a very specialized type of "skin" devoid of adnexae. It is composed of a superficial layer of **nonkeratinized stratified squamous epithelium**, that is five to eight cells thick, a superficial

(a)   (b)

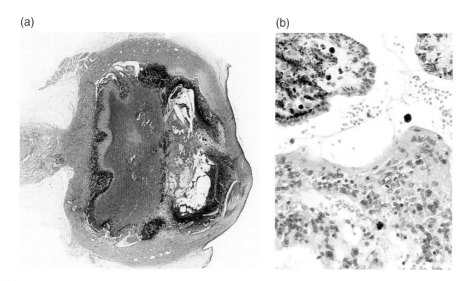

Figure 1.2   (a, b) Microphthalmia. Abnormal eye development that produces a small eye with discernible uvea and neuroepithelium that is dysplastic and disorganized.

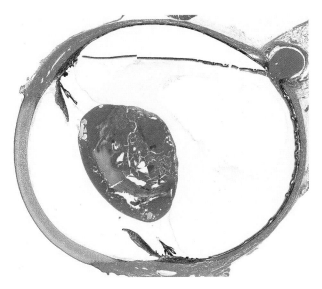

Figure 1.3　Multiple ocular defects. Abnormal development has resulted in retinal dysplasia, goniodysgenesis, and congenital cataract.

basement membrane (**Bowman's membrane**), a stroma of avascular, highly structured fibrous connective tissue, and a layer of simple squamous epithelium, referred to as **corneal endothelium**. The stroma is maintained in a relatively dehydrated state by the epithelial layers on either side; this helps preserve its organization and clarity. Between the corneal stroma and the corneal endothelium is a thick basement membrane, known as **Descemet's membrane**, which terminates at the ciliary cleft. Since the cornea is avascular, it is nourished, hydrated, and lubricated by the tear film, which is composed of secretions from the lacrimal glands and cells lining the palpebrae and conjunctiva.

General Corneal Reactions to Injury

The cornea has a limited set of reactions to various injuries that occur. Acute reactions consist of **loss of epithelium** (erosion or ulcer), **edema**, serous, fibrinous, and/or purulent inflammation, or combinations of these (Figure 1.4). When the cornea develops edema or exudate in the stroma, the organization of the collagen fibers in the stroma is perturbed, which results in cloudiness of the cornea; this is common with ulcers. Chronic reactions consist of **epithelial hyperplasia** and **keratinization**, **fibrosis** of the stroma, and **neovascularization** (Figure 1.5). Epithelial hyperplasia can become severe enough to microscopically resemble epidermis, and coupled with superficial stromal fibrosis, resemble non-haired

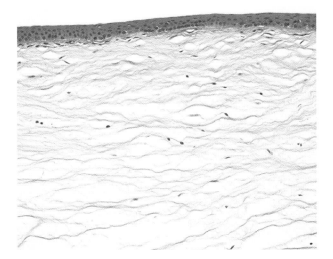

Figure 1.4　Corneal edema.

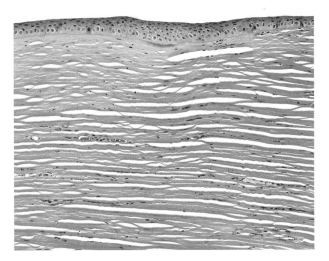

Figure 1.5 Moderate corneal stromal neovascularization.

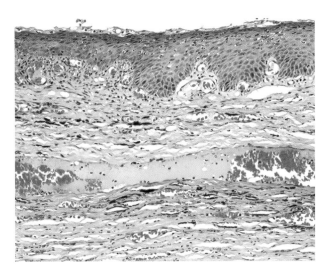

Figure 1.6 Corneal cutaneous metaplasia (epidermalization) due to chronic keratitis. There is hyperplasia with rete ridge formation of the surface epithelium. Also, there is marked fibrosis, hyperpigmentation, and neovascularization of the corneal stroma.

skin; therefore, this change is referred to as **cutaneous metaplasia** or **"epidermalization"** of the cornea (Figure 1.6). Fibrosis of the superficial stroma disrupts the normally precise organization of the stromal collagen fibers, causing corneal opacity (Figure 1.7). Neovascularization of the cornea commonly occurs secondary to ulceration, chronic keratitis, and uveitis; it will start from the limbus and progress toward the center of the cornea.

Developmental and Degenerative Corneal Disease

Corneal Dermoid
This is a developmental anomaly that consists of a patch of haired skin growing on the cornea.

Corneal Erosions and Ulcers
The loss of one or more layers of the superficial epithelium is **corneal erosion** (Figure 1.8). Loss of corneal epithelium through Bowman's membrane with exposure of the corneal stroma is an **ulcer** (Figure 1.9). These are commonly due to trauma, injury from a foreign body, or drying. In addition, ulcers are commonly associated with keratitis (corneal inflammation). Occasionally, corneal ulcers are delayed in healing because the corneal epithelium does not establish appropriate

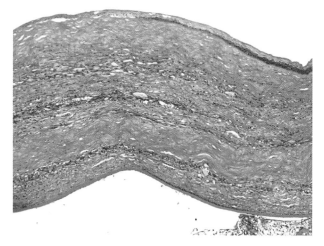

Figure 1.7 Corneal stromal fibrosis and neovascularization.

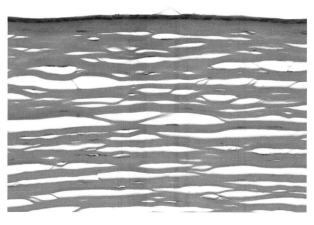

Figure 1.8 Feline corneal erosion. The surface epithelium is attenuated and only one to two layers thick.

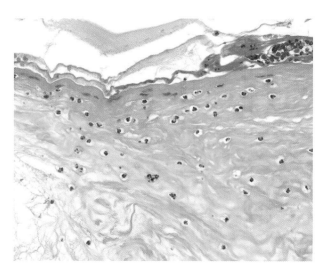

Figure 1.9 Corneal melting ulcer in a dog. The surface epithelium has been totally lost, the superficial stroma is necrotic and partially liquefied, and there are a few degenerate pmns evident.

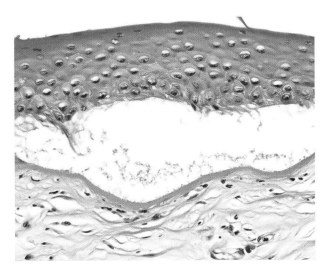

Figure 1.10 Persistent or recurring corneal ulcer. The surface epithelium regrows following ulceration but does not form hemidesmosomes for reattachment to the basement membrane, therefore ulceration recurs. Note the thickened, uneven basement membrane.

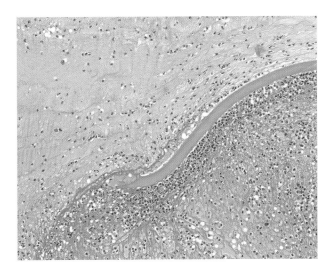

Figure 1.11 Rupture of Descemet's membrane associated with fibrinopurulent keratitis.

adhesion with the underlying basement membrane or stroma. These **persistent ulcers** occur primarily in dogs and are due to a failure of hemidesmosome production (Figure 1.10). There are several infectious agents that are noted for causing corneal ulcers in various species; **feline herpes virus** in cats is an example. A particularly deep ulcer that extends down to Descemet's membrane is very serious and will result in bulging of Descemet's membrane into the ulcer, which is called a **descemetocele**. In this condition, the cornea is in jeopardy of perforation (Figure 1.11). If the cornea does perforate, then frequently the iris will prolapse into the perforation, acting like a plug; this is a **staphyloma** (Figure 1.12a, b). Healing of corneal ulcers (depending on the depth of the ulcer) is accomplished by a combination of stromal fibrosis, re-epithelialization, and possibly neovascularization.

Corneal Sequestration
This is death of a portion of the corneal stroma, which results in a characteristic brown focus, typically in the center of the cornea (Figure 1.13). The dead tissue apparently accumulates brownish pigment from the tear film, which results in this color change. This condition almost exclusively occurs in cats, especially Persian and Himalayan cats, and is frequently associated with chronic ulceration.

(a)

(b)

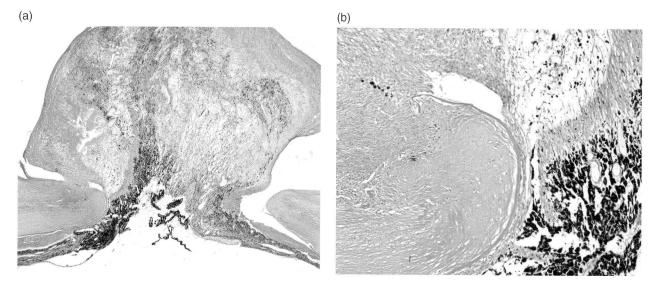

Figure 1.12   (a, b) Perforated corneal ulcer with prolapse of iris (staphyloma).

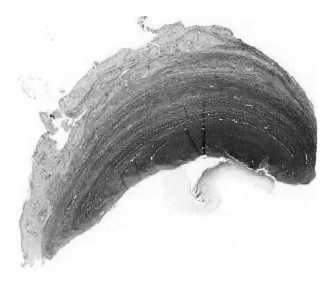

Figure 1.13   Keratectomy specimen from a cat with a corneal sequestrum. This is secondary to a chronic corneal ulcer with necrosis of the stroma. Note the characteristic brown discoloration.

Corneal Endothelial Dystrophy and Mineralization

Several breeds of dogs have a defect in corneal endothelial integrity due to degeneration, which results in seepage of aqueous humor into the corneal stroma. This results in corneal opacity due to edema (Figure 1.14a, b).

Corneal Stromal Dystrophy and Mineralization

Deposits of lipid, cholesterol, and/or mineral may occur in a variety of breeds of dogs and cats, which are recognized as specific corneal stromal dystrophies. In addition, these materials may also be deposited in the corneal stroma secondary to injury or metabolic abnormalities such as hypercholesterolemia or hypercalcemia.

Inflammatory Disease of the Cornea

Keratitis

Inflammation of the cornea is **keratitis**. As mentioned, keratitis commonly occurs with or leads to corneal ulceration (Figure 1.15). As with ulcers, keratitis also frequently is associated with abnormalities in the tear film. **Acute keratitis** is

(a)

(b)

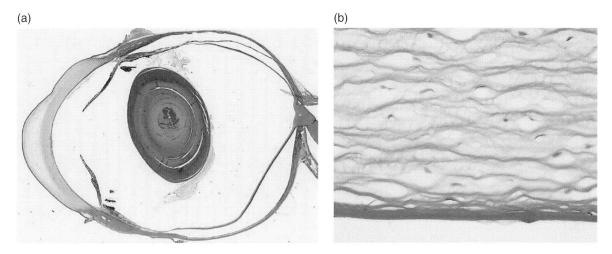

Figure 1.14   (a, b) Corneal endothelial dystrophy. There is degeneration and loss of corneal endothelium resulting in corneal edema.

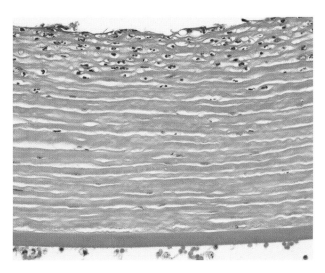

Figure 1.15   Acute ulcerative keratitis. The surface epithelium and basement membrane have been lost, and there is a moderate infiltrate of pmns within the superficial stroma.

frequently associated with conjunctivitis. Since the cornea is normally avascular, exudate that accumulates in acute keratitis must come from the tear film and adjacent vascular tissues, especially the bulbar and palpebral conjunctiva. Swelling of the cornea that occurs in acute keratitis is due to loss of epithelium and imbibition of fluid from the tear film and serous exudate from adjacent structures; this is usually referred to as "**corneal edema**" and causes the cornea to be cloudy. Neutrophils migrate into the cornea from the tear film and when numerous contribute to destruction of the corneal epithelium and stroma via the release of toxic oxidative molecules and enzymes. **Chronic keratitis** is typically characterized by neovascularization and fibrosis of the stroma with epithelial hyperplasia (Figure 1.16). Once corneal neovascularization is established, then inflammatory cells may enter the stroma through new vessels. Chronic keratitis is usually the result of a persistent injury, such as an eyelid abnormality.

Opportunistic bacteria, such as ***Pseudomonas* sp.** will occasionally colonize a small ulcer, and through production of potent enzymes that break down the stromal matrix (**matrix metaloproteinases**) and stimulate suppurative inflammation, make it much larger and progressive; this is **ulcerative and suppurative keratitis or keratomalacia** (also known as a **"melting ulcer")** (Figure 1.17a, b).

Keratitis sicca
This is chronic keratitis that develops secondary to loss of adequate tear film production or maintenance.

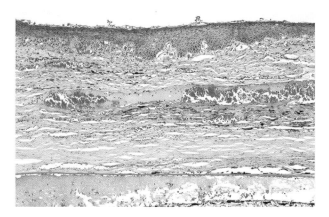

Figure 1.16   Chronic keratitis with cutaneous metaplasia. This is a common lesion that develops secondary to low-grade persistent injury associated with loss of tear film. In addition to cutaneous metaplasia, there is a moderate infiltrate of lymphocytes and plasma cells within the stroma.

(a)   (b)

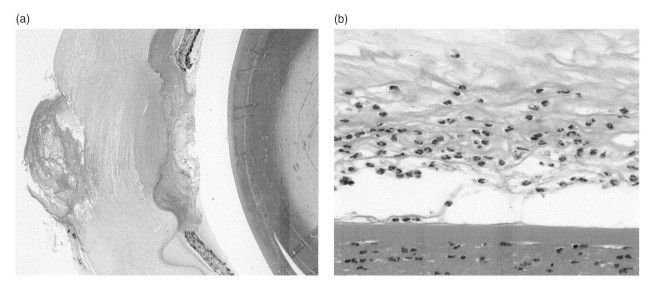

Figure 1.17   (a, b) Ulcerative and fibrinopurulent keratitis (melting ulcer). Note perforation of cornea.

Canine Pannus Keratitis (Chronic Superficial Keratitis)

This is a chronic progressive lesion that begins at the lateral limbus and spreads toward the center of the cornea. It occurs most commonly in German shepherd dogs but is not limited to this breed. Grossly, it is a red, fleshy plaque. Microscopically, it is characterized by an interface infiltrate of lymphocytes and plasma cells with vacuolar degeneration and scattered apoptosis of the basal epithelial cells, and occasionally, hyperpigmentation (Figure 1.18a, b). In addition, there is neovascularization of the superficial corneal stroma, and frequently, the superficial stroma contains scattered melanophages.

Feline Herpetic Keratitis

This disease is caused by **feline herpes virus 1 (FHV-1)**, which is characterized by corneal ulceration. There are two forms: **dendritic ulceration**, which typically involves the corneal epithelium only; and **stromal ulceration**, which is deeper, more chronic, and contains an infiltrate of lymphocytes and plasma cells.

Feline Eosinophilic Keratitis

This is a form of chronic stromal keratitis that is unique to cats. It is characterized by an inflammatory cell infiltrate of macrophages, lymphocytes, plasma cells, and few to many eosinophils (Figure 1.19). In addition, there is usually fibrosis and modest neovascularization with ulceration or hyperplasia of the overlying epithelium.

(a) (b)

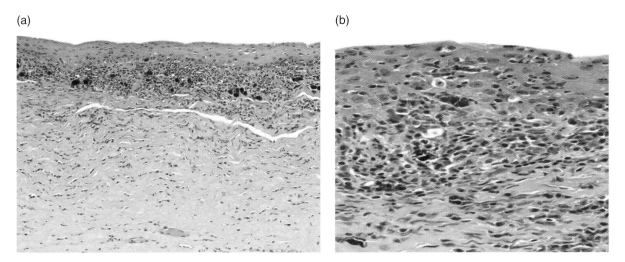

Figure 1.18   (a, b) Canine pannus keratitis (chronic superficial keratitis). There is a diffuse infiltrate of lymphocytes and plasma cells along with hyperpigmentation, pigmentary incontinence, and scattered apoptotic epithelial cells.

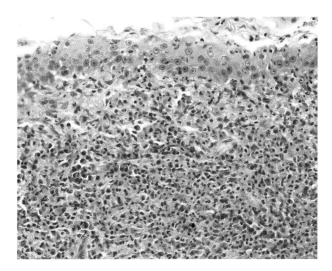

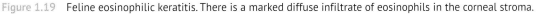

Figure 1.19   Feline eosinophilic keratitis. There is a marked diffuse infiltrate of eosinophils in the corneal stroma.

Mycotic Keratitis

Infection of the cornea with fungi is a fairly common, serious disease in horses and dogs. The agent involved is usually ***Aspergillus* sp.**, which typically enters through a corneal ulcer. *Aspergillus* sp. spreads through the corneal stroma and has a tropism for basement membrane; therefore, it typically invades the anterior basement membrane and Descemet's membrane. Fungal invasion incites a very necrotizing and fibrinopurulent reaction (Figure 1.20a–c). Occasionally, the cornea will perforate.

Equine Corneal Stromal Abscess

This is typically a collection of purulent exudate bordered by fibrovascular tissue deep in the corneal stroma (Figure 1.21a, b). Frequently, it is adjacent to Descemet's membrane. It is most likely the result of a small penetrating injury to the cornea with bacterial or fungal infection, although many times agents are not detected with histopathology.

Uvea

The uvea is composed of the **iris**, **ciliary body,** and **choroid**. It is pigmented with melanin and is very vascular. In fact, it is the main vascular supply to the outer half of the retina and provides nutrients to the lens and interior of the globe via the aqueous humor. **Aqueous humor** is an ultrafiltrate that is generated by the ciliary processes of the ciliary body and flows

(a)

(b)

(c)

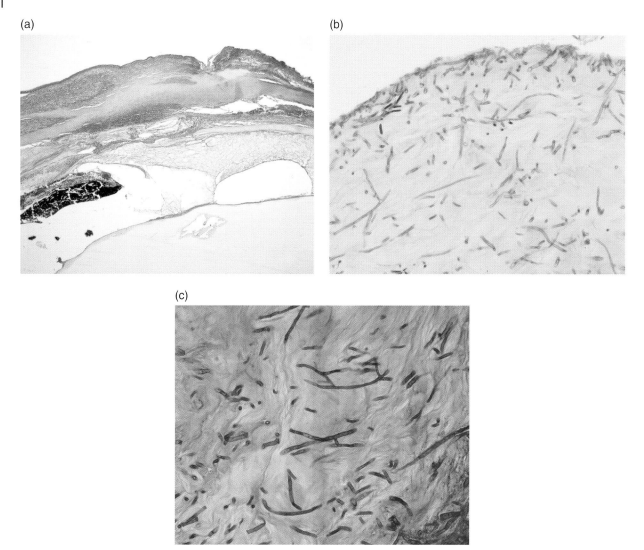

Figure 1.20 (a–c) Mycotic keratitis in a horse. There is marked ulcerative and fibrinopurulent inflammation of the cornea with fungal hyphae within the stroma.

anteriorly through the posterior chamber and pupil, into the anterior chamber, and then through the iridocorneal angle into the **ciliary cleft**. Here, aqueous humor flows into a series of interconnected vascular channels within the **trabecular meshwork** and exits the globe via scleral vessels. The iris helps regulate the amount of light passing to the lens and retina. The anterior surface of the iris is covered by a layer of melanocytes. The ciliary body is covered by epithelium, which is derived from neural tissue from the optic vesicle. The **zonular fibers** extend from the ciliary body and attach to the lens and thus hold it in place. The choroid is situated between the sclera (outside) and retina (inside). It is a fibrovascular layer, which also includes the **tapetum lucidum**. The tapetum is a reflective layer present in the dorsal portion of the globe in many mammals; it helps concentrate light for vision during relative darkness.

General Uveal Reactions to Injury

Since the uvea is a vascular structure, perhaps the most common reaction to injury is inflammation (**uveitis**). In fact, exudate that accumulates within the eye necessarily comes from the uvea and can take on various patterns that provide insight as to cause, as discussed later. **Intraocular hemorrhage** is a common lesion that can develop secondary to coagulopathy, trauma, uveitis, and intraocular neoplasms (Figure 1.22). It typically originates in the uvea, and depending on its location, may cause retinal detachment or hyphema. If severe, it will impair vision, and as it begins to organize, it will result in fibrosis that will distort intraocular structures.

(a)

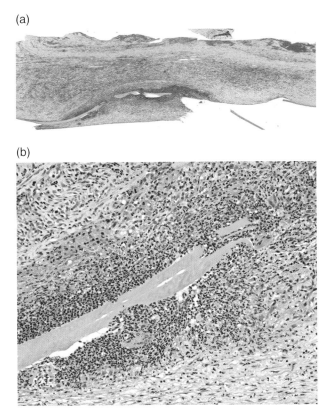

(b)

Figure 1.21   (a, b) Equine corneal abscess. En bloc removal of a deep corneal abscess in a horse.

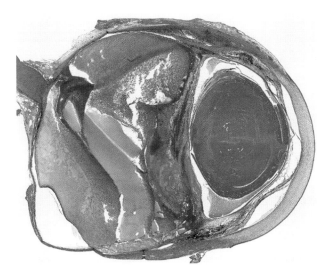

Figure 1.22   Intraocular hemorrhage filling the vitreous chamber.

Developmental and Degenerative Uveal Disease

Defective formation of the uvea during development is a common reaction to injury. Developmental defects of the uvea can vary widely in severity from mild goniodysgenesis that has little clinical significance to severe hypoplasia associated with multiple ocular defects.

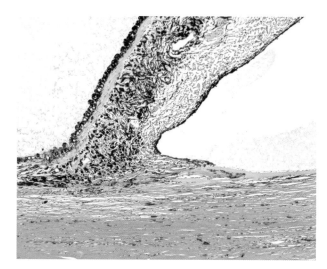

Figure 1.23 Goniodysgenesis. The termination of Descemet's membrane is split, and there is not a clearly distinct pectinate ligament or trabecular meshwork.

Goniodysgenesis and Pectinate Ligament Dysplasia

This is failure of the iridocorneal angle to develop normally. It may involve the entire circumference of the iridocorneal angle or only one or more segments (Figure 1.23). It is usually characterized by failure of the pectinate ligament to form correctly, a bulbous or abnormal termination of Descemet's membrane, failure of the ciliary cleft to open and a sheet of mesenchymal tissue in place of the trabecular meshwork. It is frequently a feature of eyes that have primary glaucoma.

Persistent Pupillary Membrane

Persistent pupillary membrane (PPM) is a developmental anomaly that is formed by the persistence of strands of the primary tunica vasculosa lentis. It is characterized by the attachment of strands of tissue (endothelial lined tubes) extending from the minor arterial circle of the iris to the cornea or anterior lens capsule. Fibrous metaplasia is usually present where these strands insert on the lens or cornea.

Choroidal Hypoplasia

This is an underdevelopment of the choroid characterized by thinning and hypopigmentation. It occurs in many species and is common in animals that have color-dilution of the hair coat. It may not be clinically significant in many instances, but it is a characteristic feature of the **Collie eye anomaly syndrome**, which is an inherited set of ocular lesions that occur in collies (Figure 1.24). The extent of the lesions may vary from case to case, but the characteristic components are choroidal hypoplasia and hypopigmentation, mild microphthalmia, scleral ectasia, and posterior coloboma adjacent to the optic nerve. The basic defect is an abnormality in RPE development, which results in failure of proper induction of the

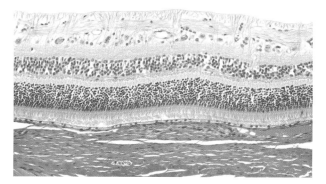

Figure 1.24 Choroidal hypoplasia in the Collie eye anomaly syndrome. The retina is fairly normal in this section, but the choroid is very thin and difficult to recognize.

(a) (b)

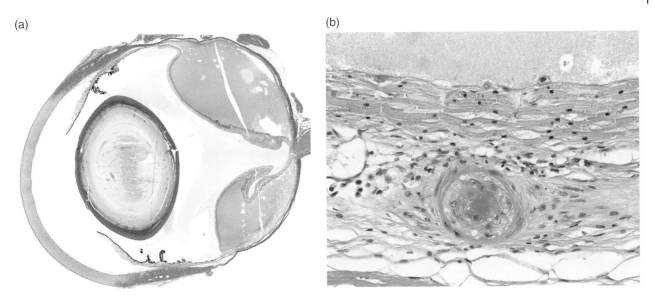

Figure 1.25 (a, b) Retinal detachment secondary to hypertensive vasculopathy in a cat with chronic renal failure.

periocular mesenchyme. This results in the failure of the choroid and sclera to develop properly and failure of the optic fissure to close properly. The retina bulges into the optic fissure, further impeding scleral development, resulting in scleral ectasia and posterior coloboma.

Hypertensive Vasculopathy

Hypertensive vasculopathy occurs in dogs and cats that have prolonged hypertension, which is frequently the result of chronic renal failure, especially in cats. The characteristic lesion is thickening and hyalinization of the walls in arterioles within the choroid and retina. This commonly leads to accumulation of transudate between the RPE and retina, resulting in retinal detachment (Figure 1.25a, b).

Inflammatory Disease of the Uvea and Ocular

Uveitis

Uveitis, inflammation of the uvea, is the most common reaction to uveal injury and is classified according to the portion of the uvea that is involved, the duration of the inflammation, and the type of exudate produced. The types of exudate that occur in uveitis vary and frequently give a clue as to the possible cause. Exudate not only is present within the uvea but may also accumulate in one or all of the ocular chambers. Most types of exudate are possible – serofibrinous, purulent, pyogranulomatous, and lymphoplasmacytic. Inflammation of the iris is **iritis**; inflammation of the ciliary body is **cyclitis**; and inflammation of the choroid is **choroiditis**. **Anterior uveitis** is inflammation of the iris and the ciliary body (also called iridocyclitis). **Panuveitis** is inflammation of all components of the uvea. **Acute uveitis** is characterized by hyperemia of the iris and the production of serous or serofibrinous exudate (and possibly pmns), which accumulates on the surface of the iris and within the anterior chamber. **Plasmoid aqueous** is a term used for the accumulation of protein from serous exudate in the aqueous humor (Figure 1.26). Accumulation of purulent exudate in the anterior chamber is **hypopyon** (Figure 1.27a, b). Occasionally exudate will adhere to the endothelial side of the cornea (the clinical term for this is **keratitic precipitates**). Injury to the corneal endothelium can result in corneal edema. An inflamed iris is prone to adhere to the endothelial surface of the cornea (**anterior synechia**) or anterior surface of the lens capsule (**posterior synechia**). Acute uveitis may resolve or progress to chronic uveitis. **Chronic uveitis** is characterized by an infiltrate of lymphocytes, plasma cells, and/or macrophages. In addition, a layer of fibrovascular tissue will frequently develop over the anterior surface of the iris; this is a **pre-iridial fibrovascular membrane (PIFM)** (Figure 1.28). **Rubeosis iridis** is the clinical term for the gross appearance of a PIFM. PIFM is a serious complication of chronic uveitis because this tissue may grow into the ciliary cleft, resulting in occlusion and secondary glaucoma. Also, PIFM may distort the pupillary margins of the iris (causing **entropion uveae** or **ectropion uveae**), cause posterior synechia with pupillary block, or anterior synechia. When

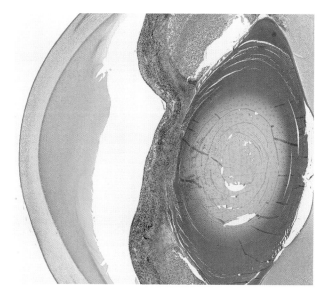

Figure 1.26 Plasmoid aqueous. This is a term used for the accumulation of protein from serous exudate in the aqueous humor. There is a marked infiltrate of lymphocytes and plasma cells in the iris.

(a)

(b)

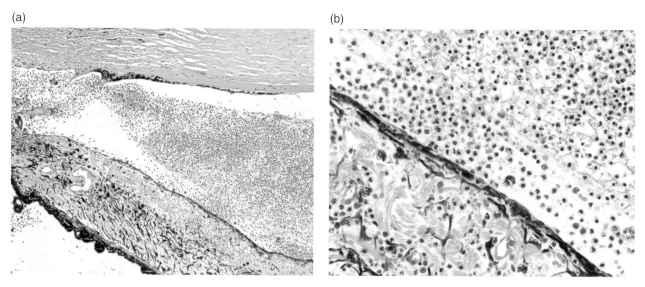

Figure 1.27 (a, b) Acute purulent anterior uveitis. The anterior chamber and ciliary cleft are filled with purulent exudate (hypopyon).

pupillary block occurs, i.e. a 360° posterior synechia, aqueous humor will accumulate in the posterior chamber, pushing against the iris; this will make the iris bulge anteriorly, a condition known as **iris bombe** (Figure 1.29). Fibrinous exudate or hemorrhage adjacent to the ciliary body will frequently be organized into a membrane that extends along the zonular fibers, covering the posterior surface of the lens; this is a **cyclitic membrane** (Figure 1.30). Another complication of chronic uveitis is the stimulation of corneal neovascularization. The end-stage inflammatory lesion of chronic uveitis or endophthalmitis is **phthisis bulbi**, which is characterized by a shrunken, fibrotic globe with partially destroyed remnants of the inner segments and lymphoplasmacytic to granulomatous exudate (Figure 1.31a, b).

Lymphoplasmacytic Anterior Uveitis

This is the most common form of uveitis in dogs, and it is usually an idiopathic condition. It is characterized by a perivascular to diffuse infiltrate of lymphocytes and plasma cells within the iris and ciliary body (Figure 1.32a, b).

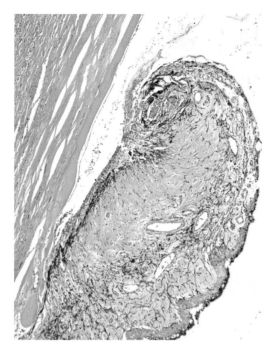

Figure 1.28   Chronic anterior uveitis with preiridial fibrovascular membrane that has distorted the iris pupillary margin (ectropion uveae) and collapsed the iridocorneal angle.

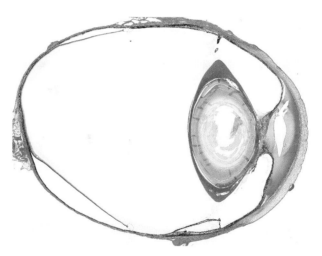

Figure 1.29   Iris bombe. Chronic anterior uveitis with a 360° posterior synechia, resulting in iris bombe. Also, the anterior chamber is filled with serofibrinous exudate and hemorrhage.

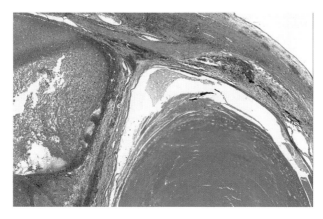

Figure 1.30   Cyclitic membrane of partially organized hemorrhage extends from the surface of the ciliary body along the posterior lens capsule.

(a)

(b)

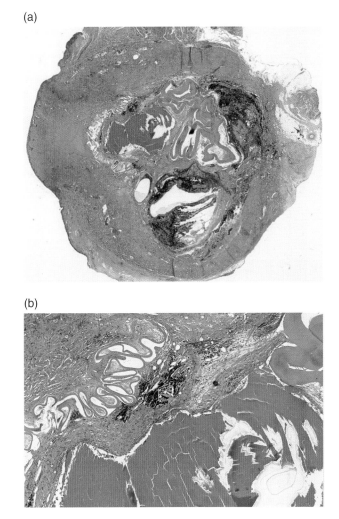

Figure 1.31   (a) Phthisis bulbi secondary to a penetrating wound through the cornea and chronic endophthalmitis. (b) Note the fibrotic cornea, convoluted Descemet's membrane, and remnants of the anterior uvea, lens capsule, and lens fibers.

(a)   (b)

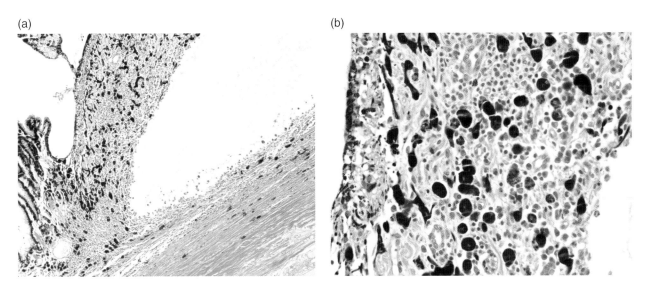

Figure 1.32   (a, b) Lymphoplasmacytic anterior uveitis. There is a diffuse infiltrate of lymphocytes and plasma cells within the iris and ciliary body that has resulted in closure of the ciliary cleft.

(a) (b)

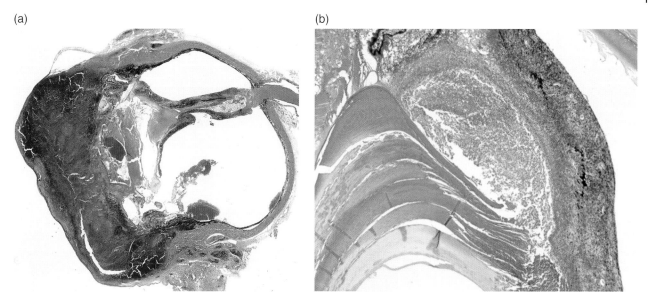

Figure 1.33 (a, b) Phacoclastic uveitis. The lens capsule has been ruptured, and the lens proteins have incited severe lymphoplasmacytic to pyogranulomatous inflammation of the uvea.

Phacoclastic Uveitis/Endophthalmitis

This is a severe form of uveitis that develops following traumatic rupture of the lens capsule. Rupture of the lens capsule allows abrupt leakage of lens proteins into the chambers of the eye, which stimulates severe inflammation within the lens (phacitis), adjacent uvea, and ocular chambers (Figure 1.33a, b). Accumulation of purulent to pyogranulomatous exudate between lens fibers, within the anterior uvea and ocular chambers, frequently with posterior synechia, is characteristic.

Phacolytic Uveitis
This is a milder form of uveitis that is caused by a less severe leakage of lens proteins, frequently secondary to maturing cataract. An infiltrate of lymphocytes and plasma cells within the anterior uvea is typical.

Equine Recurrent Uveitis
This is the most common form of uveitis in horses, and it is characterized by lymphoplasmacytic exudate with a thick layer of **amyloid-like material** covering the epithelium of the ciliary body (Figure 1.34a, b). Equine recurrent uveitis (ERU) is considered to be an autoimmune disease triggered by infection with *Leptospira* spp. The theory for the pathogenesis of ERU is that lesions occur in the uvea because it contains antigens that are similar to those on *Leptospira* sp., therefore, the immune response generated to the bacteria also targets the cross-reactive antigens in the uvea.

Uveitis Due to FIP Coronavirus
Vasculocentric pyogranulomatous and lymphoplasmacytic panuveitis are characteristic of the ocular lesions that occur in **feline infectious peritonitis** (Figure 1.35a–c). This is an important multisystem disease that is caused by infection with a feline coronavirus (FIP virus) and the profound, yet ineffective immune reaction to this virus. The disease develops in cats that are unable to clear the virus but continually mount an ineffective immune response to the virus. The eyes are a common location for lesions with FIP.

Canine Uveodermatologic Syndrome (VKH-like Syndrome)
This is an autoimmune disease that occurs in dogs, primarily in Akitas, Samoyeds, and Siberian Huskies, which targets the pigmented segments of the eye and skin. This results in **severe granulomatous panuveitis/endophthalmitis** and **interface dermatitis** (Figure 1.36a, b).

(a)

(b)

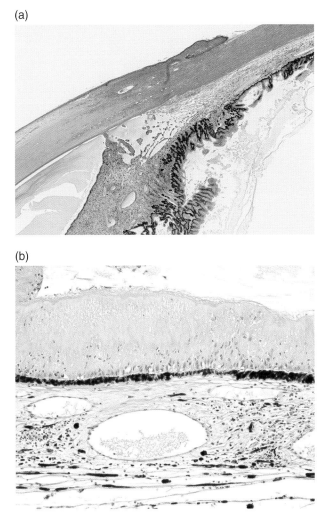

Figure 1.34 (a, b) Equine recurrent uveitis. There is serous exudate in the anterior chamber along with a perivascular to diffuse infiltrate of lymphocytes and plasma cells in the iris and ciliary body. Also there is amyloid-like material covering the neuroepithelium of the ciliary body.

Pigmentary Uveitis

This is a condition that occurs primarily in Golden Retrievers and is characterized by multiple thin-walled uveal cysts, usually on the ciliary body and posterior surface of the iris (Figure 1.37a, b). In addition, there is substantial melanin pigment throughout the anterior chamber, vitreous, ciliary cleft, trabecular meshwork, and adhered to the lens capsule. However, there is only a minimal inflammatory infiltrate in the uvea. This results in cataract and secondary glaucoma.

Endophthalmitis and Panophthalmitis

Endophthalmitis is not a specific disease but is an inflammatory condition of the eye characterized by **inflammation of all interior segments and chambers of the eye**. Typically exudate is present within the anterior, posterior, and vitreous chambers. **Panophthalmitis** is essentially endophthalmitis plus inflammation of the sclera and cornea. The character of the exudate can vary from serous to granulomatous, but usually it includes fibrin and pmns. When serofibrinous exudate is grossly evident in the aqueous and/or vitreous chambers, it is referred to as **plasmoid aqueous** or **plasmoid vitreous**, respectively. Endophthalmitis and/or panophthalmitis are characteristic of several diseases, including blastomycosis, cryptococcosis, feline infectious peritonitis, and intraocular bacterial infections, especially those from corneal perforation or penetrating foreign objects.

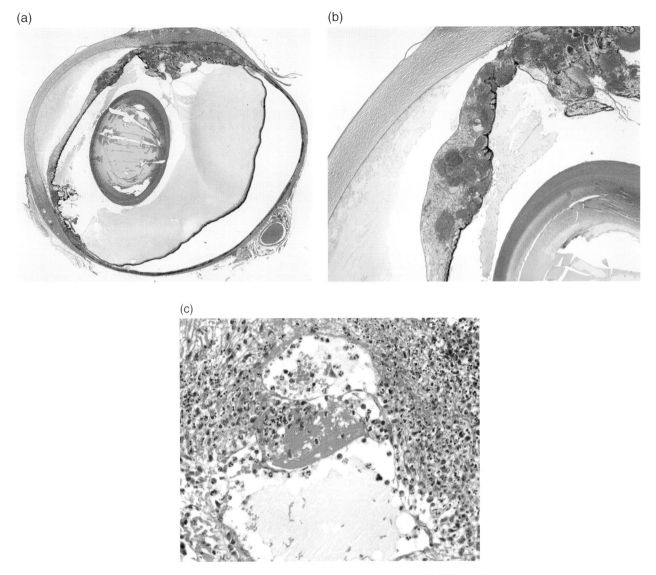

Figure 1.35 (a–c) Feline infectious peritonitis-associated panuveitis. The eye lesion with FIP is typically a lymphoplasmacytic to pyogranulomatous vasculocentric infiltrate in the iris, ciliary body, and choroid.

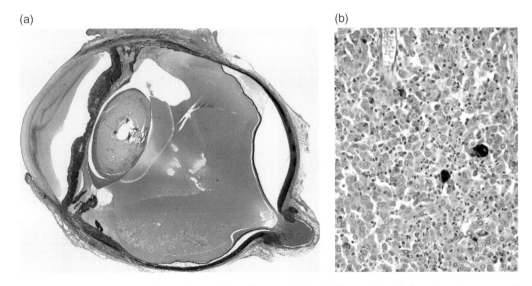

Figure 1.36 (a, b) Canine uveodermatologic syndrome (Vogt–Koyanagi–Harada-like syndrome). Granulomatous panuveitis/endophthalmitis focused on the melanocytes within the eye.

(a) (b)

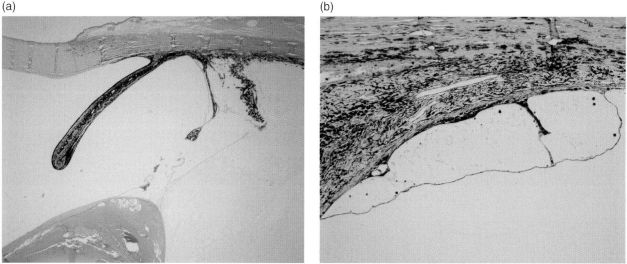

Figure 1.37   (a, b) Pigmentary uveitis is characterized by proliferation of melanin-containing cells throughout the uvea, along with multiple thin-walled uveal cysts.

Bacterial Endophthalmitis

Intraocular bacterial infections can occur from blood-borne pathogens or from a wound, especially those from a perforated corneal ulcer or a penetrating foreign object. Hematogenous intraocular infection most commonly occurs in neonatal animals, especially those with failure of passive transfer of maternal immunity. Intraocular bacterial infection from a penetrating wound is the more common route in enucleated eyes submitted for pathologic evaluation. In these eyes, there is commonly a mixed population of bacteria, both bacilli and cocci. The infection spreads throughout the eye, and all chambers are typically filled with purulent or fibrinopurulent exudate (Figure 1.38a–c).

Ocular Blastomycosis

Blastomycosis is a disease caused by the yeast form of the dimorphic fungus *Blastomyces dermatitidis*. It is typically a systemic disease in dogs that frequently involves the lungs, bones, lymph nodes, eyes, and a variety of other organs. The characteristic lesion, regardless of the organ involved, is pyogranulomatous inflammation centered on one or more organisms. In microscopic sections, the yeasts are round, have a thick refractile wall, are 15–30 μm in diameter, and replicate via broad-based budding (Figure 1.39a, b). Ocular involvement has a characteristic distribution in which organisms and associated pyogranulomatous exudate first accumulate in the choroid and subretinal space, and then spread into the retina and vitreous chamber; occasionally, inflammation may extend through the sclera. The anterior uvea is frequently inflamed; however, organisms rarely are found in the anterior chamber or iris. Since the interior segments of the eye (uvea, retina) and all chambers (vitreous, posterior, aqueous) are involved, this becomes endophthalmitis; if the cornea and sclera are also involved, then it becomes panophthalmitis.

Ocular Cryptococcosis

Cryptococcosis is another disease caused by yeast, similar to blastomycosis. *Cryptococcus neoformans* is the agent; it is an oval to spherical yeast that is 5–20 μm in diameter and surrounded by a thick mucinous capsule, which produces a clear zone around the yeast in microscopic sections. This may be a systemic disease, but also it is commonly limited to the nasal cavity, brain, and eyes in dogs and cats. The distribution within the eyes is similar to blastomycosis, although the reaction is more purely granulomatous with few pmns but numerous macrophages surrounding yeasts (Figure 1.40a, b).

Ocular Coccidioidomycosis

Coccidioidomycosis induces granulomatous to pyogranulomatous inflammation that primarily starts in the choroid. The yeast form of *Coccidioides immitis* replicates by endosporulation, forming spherules that are much larger than the other yeasts found within the eye. Organisms range up to 50 μm in diameter and have a double-refractile wall.

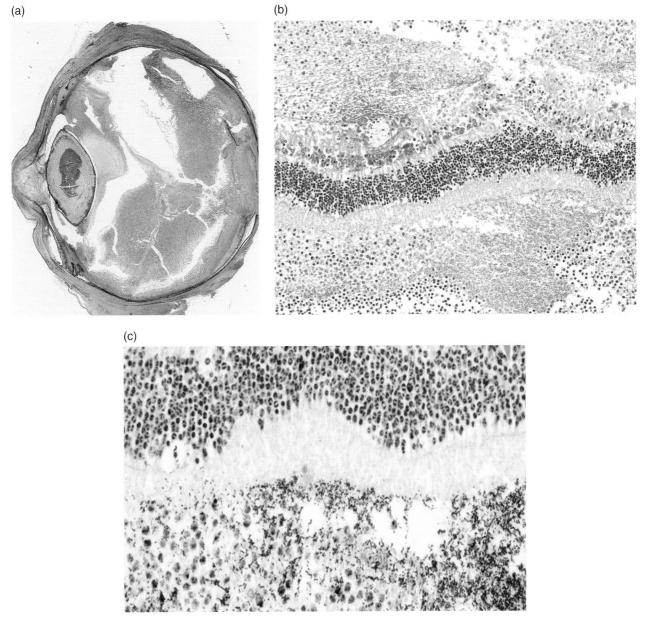

Figure 1.38   (a, b) Purulent endophthalmitis caused by an intraocular bacterial infection. There is inflammation of the interior segments of the eye with accumulation of exudate within all chambers. (c) Gram + coccoid bacteria.

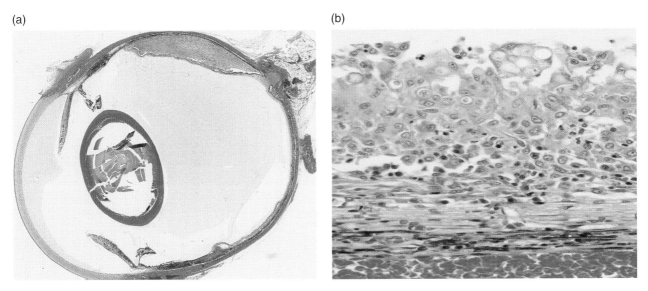

Figure 1.39   (a, b) Ocular blastomycosis. The characteristic lesion seen here is granulomatous exudate along with yeasts within the choroid and subretinal space. Also, there is serofibrinous exudate within the anterior, posterior and vitreous chambers.

(a)　　　　　　　　　　　　　　　　　　(b)

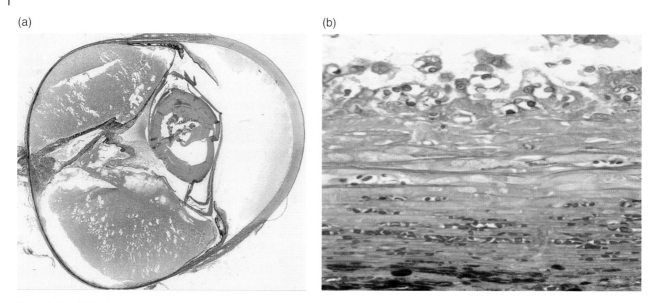

Figure 1.40　(a) Ocular cryptococcosis in a cat. The characteristic lesion is accumulation of exudate and yeasts within the choroid and subretinal space. There is marked retinal detachment as a result of exudate accumulation in the subretinal space. (b) PAS stain demonstrates yeasts.

Ocular Histoplasmosis

Histoplasmosis induces granulomatous inflammation that also starts in the choroid. Macrophages contain clusters of *Histoplasma capsulatum*, which are 2–4 μm diameter yeasts.

Ocular Prototheccosis

Prototheccosis is an uncommon disease that can involve the eyes in dogs. It is caused by one of two *Prototheca* sp., which are colorless alga. The organism is round to oval, 5–20 μm in diameter and replicates by endosporulation. The daughter cells number from 2 to 20, are wedge-shaped and remain within the cell wall of the parent cell. The cleavage lines between daughter cells form a variety of patterns, such as crosses, "Y"s and stars. The inflammatory reaction and distribution within the eye is similar to the intra-ocular dimorphic fungal infections: granulomatous exudate surrounding numerous organisms primarily in the choroid, subretinal space, and vitreous chamber (Figure 1.41a, b).

(a)　　　　　　　　　　　　　　　　　　(b)

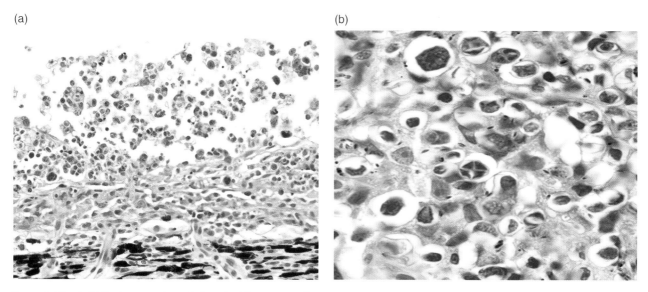

Figure 1.41　(a, b) Ocular prototheccosis in a dog. The pattern of granulomatous inflammation is similar to intraocular dimorphic fungal infections, such as blastomycosis. The organism is round to oval, 5–20 μm in diameter and replicate by endosporulation. The daughter cells number from 2 to 20, are wedge-shaped and remain within the cell wall of the parent cell. The cleavage lines between daughter cells form a variety of patterns, such as crosses, "Y"s, and stars.

Lens

The lens is composed of epithelium surrounded by a basement membrane, the lens capsule. It is held in place between the iris (anterior) and the vitreous body (posterior) by zonular fibers from the ciliary body. The epithelium under the anterior surface of the lens capsule contains germinative cells that replicate throughout life. These epithelial cells migrate posteriorly and centrally, elongate, and become lens fibers. Also, over the years, lens fibers will compress centrally, forming the lens nucleus. In addition, as an animal ages, the anterior lens capsule will progressively thicken.

General Lens Reactions to Injury

The lens is a tough, durable structure, and it takes a significant injury to damage an otherwise healthy lens. There are a limited number of reactions to injury that occur, which include rupture of the capsule, epithelial fibrous metaplasia, mineralization, cataract, and inflammation. The subcapsular lens epithelium may proliferate and undergo **fibrous metaplasia** in response to injury to the capsule or posterior synechia (Figure 1.42). This change will interfere with the clarity of the lens. Injury to the lens epithelium from a variety of causes can result in cataract, which causes lens opacity and is discussed in more detail below. Ocular trauma or a penetrating foreign object may cause **rupture of the lens capsule**; this typically results in the inflammation of the lens (phacitis) and phacoclastic uveitis, as previously discussed (Figure 1.43).

Lens Luxation

Occasionally, the lens will break loose from its attachment sites and be displaced, usually anteriorly. This can result in pupillary block and acute glaucoma. Certain breeds of dogs, especially terriers, are prone to spontaneous lens luxation because they have somewhat weak zonules. Also, lens luxation can occur secondary to trauma or be a complication of buphthalmos. A luxated lens may occlude the pupil, causing pupillary block and secondary glaucoma.

Developmental and Degenerative Disease of the Lens

Microphakia and Aphakia

These are developmental defects that result in absence of a lens (aphakia) or a lens that is smaller than normal (microphakia) (Figure 1.44). Microphakia is the more common lesion, and it is usually associated with **multiple ocular anomalies**. It is common for microphakic lenses to also have congenital cataract.

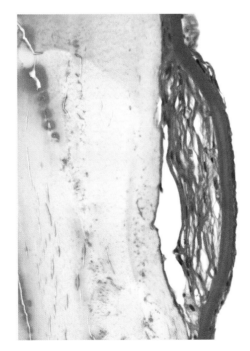

Figure 1.42 Fibrous metaplasia of the subcapsular lens epithelium secondary to injury of the capsule.

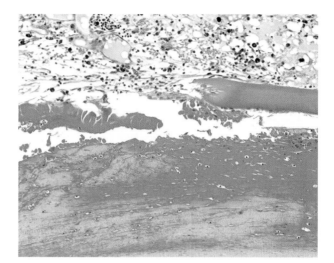

Figure 1.43   Rupture of the lens capsule with associated uveitis and phacitis.

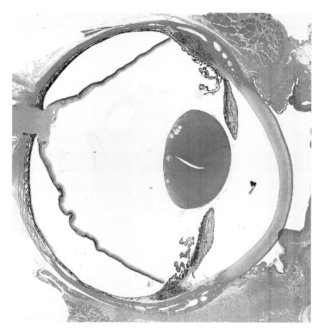

Figure 1.44   Microphakia with congenital cataract and retinal dysplasia.

Persistent Pupillary Membrane, Persistent Primary (Hyperplastic) Vitreous, Persistent Posterior Tunica Vasculosa Lentis, and Persistent Hyaloid Artery

These are developmental anomalies due to the persistence of remnants of the embryonal vascular and mesenchymal structure surrounding and supplying the lens, the **primary vitreous**. The vascular tunic around the lens, which is a subcomponent of the primary vitreous, is the **tunica vasculosa lentis.** Anomalies of these structures commonly occur with other developmental anomalies, such as microphthalmia, microphakia, and congenital cataract. **PPM** is characterized by the attachment of strands of tissue (endothelial lined tubes) extending from the minor arterial circle of the iris to the cornea or anterior lens capsule. Fibrous metaplasia is usually present where these strands insert on the lens or cornea. **PPV** or **PPHV** is characterized by a cord of vascular tissue and associated extracellular matrix extending from the optic disc to and covering the posterior lens capsule. **PPTVL** is characterized by a residual band of fibrovascular tissue along the posterior lens capsule (Figure 1.45a, b). In the developing eye, the **hyaloid artery** extends from the optic disk to the tunica vasculosa lentis on the posterior surface of the lens. Occasionally, remnants of this vessel will persist (Figure 1.46).

(a)   (b)

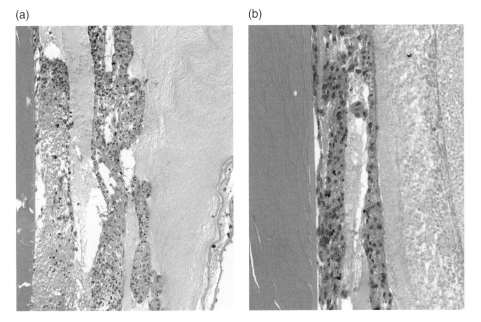

Figure 1.45   (a, b) Persistent primary tunica vasculosa lentis. This is a remnant of the embryonal vascular tunic that surrounds the lens. The PPTVL is adhered to the posterior lens capsule, which is on the left in this slide.

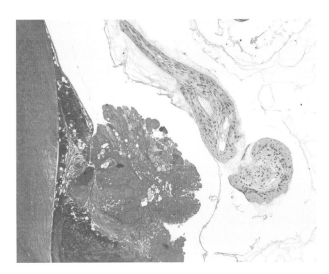

Figure 1.46   Persistent hyaloid artery and congenital cataract.

Cataract

Opacity of the lens is known as **cataract** (Figure 1.47). There are several different causes for cataracts, but the microscopic changes that occur are similar for all. Injury to the lens fibers results in the hydropic degeneration and swelling with the production of **bladder cells** (Figure 1.48). Denatured cytoplasm from the injured fibers is liberated and forms eosinophilic globules, known as **Morgagnian globules** (Figure 1.49). Also, degenerate lens fibers may fragment, liquefy, and/or mineralize. Certain types of cataracts have a genetic basis, others may be due to accumulated injury over many years, and still others are due to abnormality in lens metabolism. Cataracts that occur in **diabetes mellitus** are an example of the latter. When dogs are hyperglycemic due to DM, glucose accumulates within the lens fibers and is converted to sorbitol. Sorbitol will osmotically attract water, and therefore, the lens fibers swell (hydropic degeneration); this results in lens opacity.

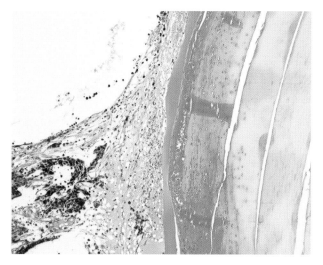

Figure 1.47 Posterior synechiae with cortical cataract.

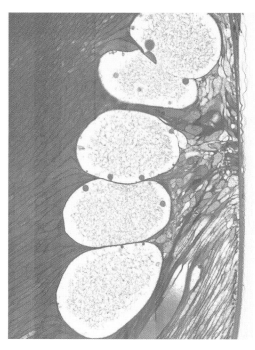

Figure 1.48 Congenital cataract with swollen lens fiber.

Sometimes a cataract will totally liquefy and only the lens capsule and liquefied lens fibers remain; this is called a "**hypermature cataract**" (Figure 1.50).

Phacitis

Inflammation of the lens is **phacitis** (Figure 1.51a, b). It usually occurs when there has been a penetrating injury through the lens capsule. Exudate, usually pmns, will accumulate under the perforated capsule and dissect between lens fibers. Abrupt leakage of lens proteins can result in a severe form of uveitis, **phacoclastic uveitis**, which was previously described. A less severe form of uveitis, **phacolytic uveitis**, may occur when lens proteins slowly leak from the lens.

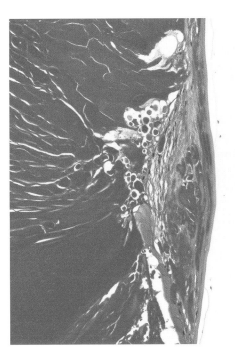

Figure 1.49   Cortical cataract with fibrous metaplasia of lens epithelium along with fragmented lens fibers and liberated lens proteins forming Morgagnian globules.

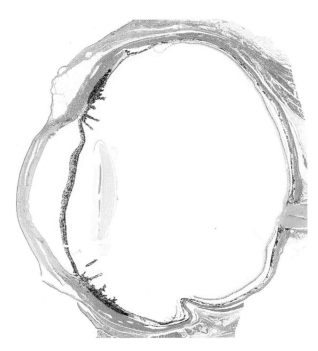

Figure 1.50   Hypermature cataract. The lens fibers are totally degenerate and liquefied. The lens shrinks, clears, and may leave only the capsule.

Retina

The retina is the neurosensory portion of the eye. It is derived from the optic vesicle, which is an extension from the brain. It is composed of eight distinct layers, from the innermost layer to the outermost layer: these are nerve fiber layer, ganglion cell layer, inner plexiform layer, inner nuclear layer, outer plexiform layer, outer nuclear layer, photoreceptor layer, and

(a)　　　　　　　　　　　　　　　　　　　　(b)

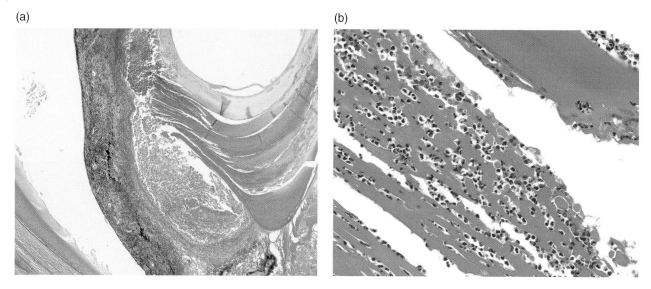

Figure 1.51　(a, b) Phacitis and phacoclastic uveitis secondary to rupture of the lens capsule. Note the pmns between the degenerate lens fibers.

RPE. The retina is only attached at its periphery (ora ciliaris retinae) and at the optic nerve head; it is held in place against the choroid by the vitreous body. The retina has its own blood supply, which enters through the optic nerve.

General Retinal Reactions to Injury

Degeneration, atrophy, inflammation, and glial scarring are the typical reactions to injury that occur in the retina. **Retinal degeneration (RD)** is best defined as loss of one or more retinal components, usually neural, as a result of injury. RD may occur as a primary disease, or it may develop secondary to other ocular diseases, such as glaucoma. RD can occur in several patterns and can be due to a variety of causes; the pattern of degeneration can indicate the cause. The patterns of RD are due to the segment(s) of the retina affected. The inner segments (ganglion cells and inner nuclear layer) can be preferentially affected compared to the outer segments (outer nuclear layer and photoreceptors); this is typical of **RD due to glaucoma**. Conversely, the outer segments may be preferentially affected, which is typical of **nutritionally-induced or inherited types of RD**. In certain diseases, such as glaucoma, the tapetal retina is preferentially spared (**tapetal-sparing effect**) from degeneration compared to the nontapetal retina. Specific cellular changes that occur in RD include acute neuronal swelling, acute neuronal necrosis resulting in loss of neurons, and loss of photoreceptors. There are a variety of causes for RD; these include too much light, inherited RD, specific nutritional deficiencies (vitamin A, taurine in cats), increased intraocular pressure, ischemia, and retinal detachment. **Retinal atrophy** is more or less the end stage of retinal degeneration or retinitis, when there has been such extensive loss of retinal components that the retina is thin, hypocellular, and gliotic. Primary **retinitis** is not a common lesion in surgical specimens, but may occur with certain neurotropic viral infections and along with uveitis and endophthalmitis.

Developmental and Degenerative Retinal Disease

Retinal Dysplasia
Dysplasia is a developmental abnormality that is characterized by folds, wrinkles, or rosettes in the retina. This is the result of injury to the developing retina. There are several recognized syndromes, such as the **skeletal-ocular dysplasia syndrome of Labrador retrievers**, in which retinal dysplasia is a component of an inherited disease with multiple ocular anomalies (Figure 1.52a, b).

Lysosomal Storage Diseases
These are a group of rare diseases in which a specific enzyme is deficient, resulting in failure of a metabolic pathway that allows intracellular accumulation of a substrate. In companion animals, these are inherited enzyme deficiencies. Affected

(a)
(b)

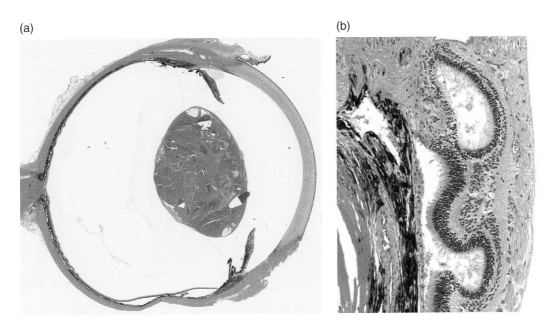

Figure 1.52 (a, b) Retinal dysplasia and congenital cataract. Retinal dysplasia is characterized by folds, wrinkles, and/or rosette-like structures.

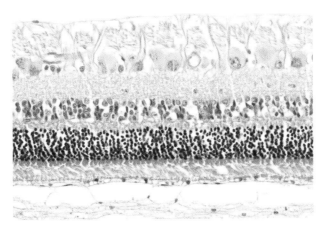

Figure 1.53 GM1 gangliosidosis. This is an example of a lysosomal storage disease in which incompletely metabolized substrate accumulates within ganglion neurons of the retina.

cells will become engorged with the substrate resulting in enlargement, vacuolization, and dysfunction. Since neurons are long-lived cells and frequently contain the dysfunctional pathway, they commonly have lesions. Neurons in the retina, especially ganglion cells, are frequently affected (Figure 1.53).

Cystic Retinal Degeneration

This occurs at the ora ciliaris retinae and is a common incidental lesion in older dogs (Figure 1.54).

Inherited Retinal Dysplasia and/or Degeneration (Progressive Retinal Atrophy)

This is a group of inherited retinal diseases that result in loss of rods, cones, or both and ultimately, neurons from the outer nuclear layer. One disease in this group is rod and cone dysplasia of Irish setter dogs. In this condition, the rods and cones do not develop normally due to a defect in the enzyme that breaks down cGMP (a phosphodiesterase). There are conditions in

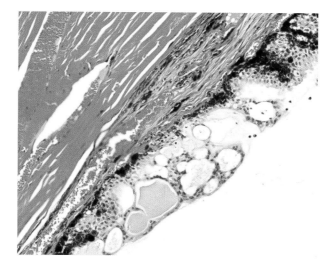

Figure 1.54   Cystic retinal degeneration. This is a common incidental aging lesion that occurs at the ora ciliaris retinae in dogs.

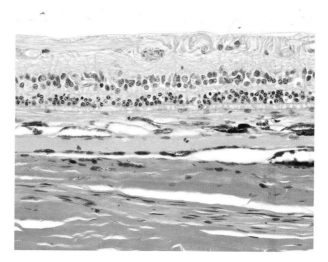

Figure 1.55   Progressive retinal atrophy (inherited retinal dysplasia/degeneration) in a Pug. The retina is thin due to hypocellularity of the outer nuclear layer and loss of the photoreceptor layer.

other breeds, in which the rods and cones develop normally, but begin to degenerate within a few years. The net result is atrophy of the retina, especially the central retina, due to loss of photoreceptors and neurons from the outer nuclear layer (Figure 1.55).

Nutritionally Induced Retinopathy

Several dietary deficiencies will cause retinal degeneration, including deficiencies of vitamin A and E. In companion animals, deficiency of the amino acid taurine is a notable cause of retinal degeneration in cats. The retinal lesion from **taurine deficiency** is degeneration of the outer nuclear and photoreceptor layers in the central area of the retina (Figure 1.56).

Toxic Retinopathy

This is not particularly common in companion animals. However, **enrofloxacin**, a widely used fluoroquinolone antibiotic, will cause retinal degeneration in cats, especially those receiving prolonged treatment. The resulting retinal lesion is thinning of the retina due to loss of the outer nuclear and photoreceptor layers, similar to taurine deficiency.

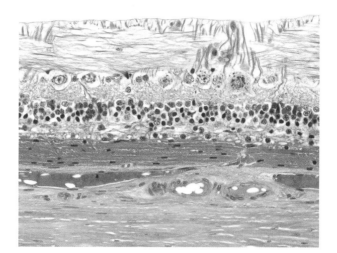

Figure 1.56   Retinopathy in a cat due to dietary taurine deficiency. There is diffuse loss of the photoreceptor layer and outer nuclear layer.

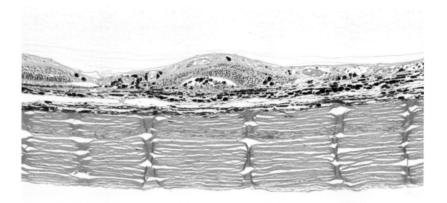

Figure 1.57   Multifocal retinal scars due to retinal ischemia and infarction. In the scarred areas of the retina, there is loss of all layers with replacement by glia and melanophages.

Ischemic and Infarctive Retinopathy

Retinal ischemia resulting in infarction can have a variety of causes including systemic thrombotic disease (DIC), vasculitis, hypertension, retinal detachment, and intra-ocular neoplasms. The acute retinal lesion that results is coagulative necrosis proceeds to liquefaction, much like necrosis in the brain. If the animal survives long enough for these lesions to heal, then one or more retinal scars will form, which are characterized by a thin, collapsed gliotic focus that lacks identifiable retinal layers and contains an accumulation of melanophages derived from injury to the RPE (Figure 1.57).

Glaucoma

Glaucoma is a disease characterized by increased intraocular pressure. It can be classified in several different ways, but the two main classifications are primary glaucoma and secondary glaucoma. Glaucoma can also be classified as open or closed-angle glaucoma, depending upon whether or not the iridocorneal angle is open (and looks normal) or closed. Primary glaucoma, as the name indicates, is glaucoma that occurs without any antecedent disease. Secondary glaucoma is an increase in intraocular pressure secondary to some other intraocular disease, such as uveitis. Primary glaucoma occurs preferentially in certain breeds of dogs, such as Basset hounds and cocker spaniels. Frequently, primary glaucoma is associated with abnormal development of the pectinate ligament, ciliary cleft, and trabecular meshwork; this is called goniodysgenesis. With goniodysgenesis, the flow of aqueous humor through the ciliary cleft is somewhat impeded, which leads to elevated IO pressure. Secondary glaucoma is usually caused by some process that closes or collapses the ciliary cleft. In primary or secondary, open or closed-angle glaucoma, the net result is the same. Increased IO pressure results in degeneration and atrophy of the

(a)

(b)

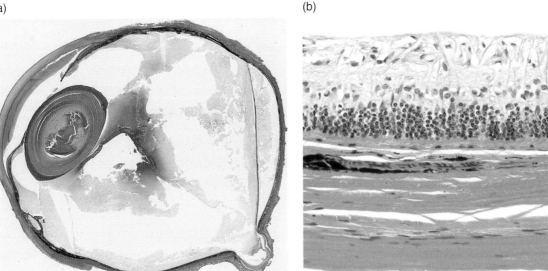

(c)

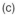

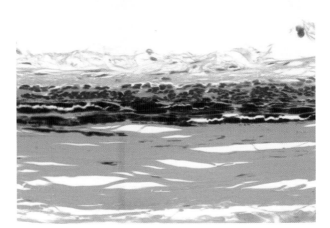

Figure 1.58 (a) Glaucoma secondary to uveitis. The iridocorneal angle is closed, and there is posterior synechia. Characteristic lesions of chronic glaucoma include buphthalmos, retinal degeneration, and cupping of the optic disk. (b, c) Characteristic retinal lesions are loss of the nerve fiber layer, ganglion neurons, inner nuclear layer neurons, and plexiform layers (left photo). The outer nuclear layer and photoreceptor layers are relatively spared until late in the disease. Retinal atrophy is the last stage of glaucoma.

inner layers (especially the ganglion and inner nuclear layers) of the retina, and eventually cupping of the optic nerve head. In addition, the increased in IO pressure is painful and frequently causes enlargement of the globe (buphthalmos) (Figure 1.58a–c). This can result in failure of the eyelids to cover the cornea and maintain an adequate tear film, thus leading to drying and chronic keratitis.

Sudden Acquired Retinal Degeneration Syndrome
This is an idiopathic disease that can affect any dog, young or old, which is characterized by a very rapid onset of blindness due to acute bilateral diffuse degeneration of the rods and cones, progressing to apoptosis of photoreceptor cells of the outer nuclear layer, and eventually loss of neurons in the inner retinal segments (Figure 1.59). Another similar syndrome, cancer-associated retinopathy, occasionally occurs in dogs with cancer; the microscopic lesions of which are similar to those in sudden acquired retinal degeneration syndrome (SARDS).

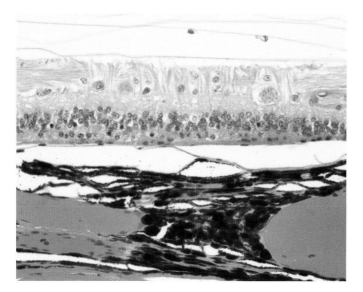

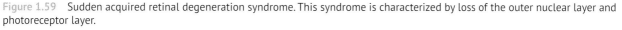

Figure 1.59 Sudden acquired retinal degeneration syndrome. This syndrome is characterized by loss of the outer nuclear layer and photoreceptor layer.

Retinal Detachment

Since the retina is only attached at the optic nerve head and the ora ciliaris retinae, sometimes it becomes pathologically separated from the adjacent tissue in the globe, and this is known as **retinal detachment**. The separation actually occurs within the retina – between the photoreceptor layer and the RPE. This is usually the result of one of the following: loss of the vitreous body, anterior traction on the retina due to intraocular hemorrhage, or accumulation of edema fluid, exudate, or hemorrhage in the subretinal space (Figure 1.60). Once the retina is detached, the outer segments of the retina, especially the photoreceptors, will begin to degenerate. Foci of retinal necrosis may develop. Also, the RPE will hypertrophy and resemble a row of little tombstones (Figure 1.61a, b).

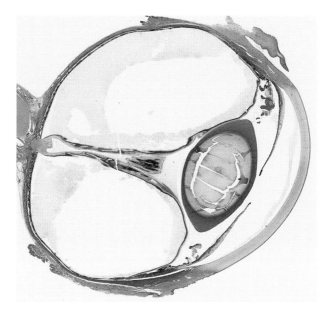

Figure 1.60 Retinal detachment in a dog with hypertension due to chronic renal failure. Serous fluid accumulates in the subretinal space secondary to hypertensive vasculopathy in the choroid.

(a) (b)

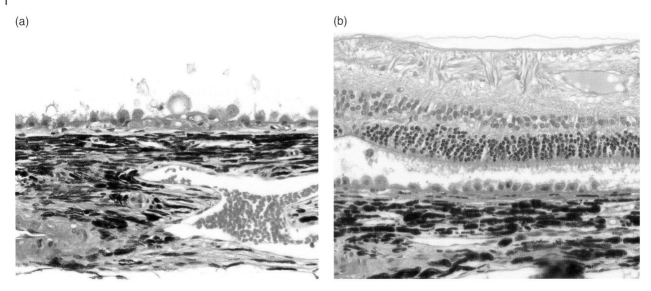

Figure 1.61 (a, b) Retinal pigment epithelium hypertrophy. There may be multiple causes for retinal detachment, but hypertrophy of the retinal pigment epithelium along with degeneration and loss of photoreceptors are characteristic changes of detachment due to any cause.

Inflammatory Disease of the Retina

Retinitis

Retinitis is inflammation of the retina. Although any type of exudate is possible, retinitis is usually characterized by a perivascular infiltrate of lymphocytes and/or plasma cells. Retinitis alone is fairly uncommon; it usually accompanies inflammation in the uvea, especially the choroid; however, some neurotropic viral infections, such as canine distemper, may localize in the retina and cause lymphocytic retinitis.

Optic Nerve

The optic nerve, cranial nerve II, is the mature structure derived from the stalk portion of the optic vesicle. Histologically, it is essentially an extension of the white matter from the brain and does not resemble peripheral or other cranial nerves. It is composed of myelinated axons that come from the ganglion neurons and nerve fiber layer of the retina. Within the globe, it begins as the optic disk, then exits the globe through the sclera at the lamina cribosa and is surrounded by the meninges. The right and left optic nerves meet at the optic chiasm before entering the brain.

Developmental and Degenerative Disease of the Optic Nerve

Hypoplasia of the Optic Nerve and/or Optic Chiasm

This may be the result of prenatal injury to the developing globe and/or skull, as caused by vitamin A deficiency or a variety of teratogens. Hypoplasia of the optic nerve may be associated with microphthalmia but is otherwise rarely seen in surgical pathology specimens.

Axonal Degeneration and Atrophy of the Optic Nerve

This is more common than hypoplasia and is typically caused by chronic injury from an adjacent expanding mass (such as a retrobulbar meningioma), ischemia, or long-standing glaucoma. Microscopic features include swelling of degenerate axons (spheroids), dilated axon sheaths containing axonal and myelin debris, gitter cells, and an increased number of activated astrocytes (Figure 1.62).

Cavitation of Optic Disk

Cavitation or cupping of the optic disk is a lesion that develops secondary to prolonged intraocular pressure and is indicative of long-standing glaucoma. In addition, microscopic changes usually associated with cavitation are axonal degeneration, myelin loss, and astrogliosis (Figure 1.63).

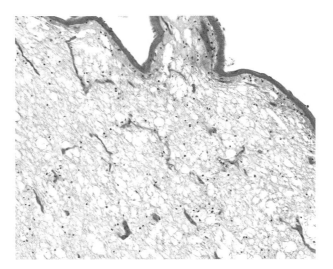

Figure 1.62 Axonal degeneration of the optic nerve characterized by numerous dilated axon sheaths.

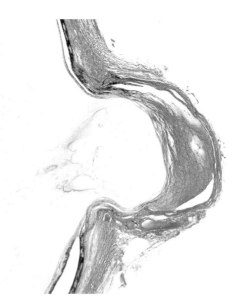

Figure 1.63 Cavitation of the optic disk due to glaucoma.

Canine Ocular Gliovascular Syndrome

This is a somewhat unusual set of lesions that primarily affects the optic disk. The optic disk is gliotic and covered with a layer of fibrovascular tissue and glial cells that protrudes into the vitreous chamber. In addition, there are usually several secondary lesions, including PIFM formation with the closure of the iridocorneal angle and secondary glaucoma. Canine ocular gliovascular syndrome (COGS) may occur more commonly in Labrador Retrievers (Figure 1.64a, b).

Inflammatory Disease of the Optic Nerve

Optic Neuritis

Inflammation of the optic nerve is not a particularly common lesion but will occasionally occur secondary to infection with agents that commonly infect the CNS. Examples would include canine distemper virus, arboviruses (EEE, WEE, West Nile), and aberrantly migrating ascarids (*Baylisascaris* sp., *Toxacara* sp.). With canine distemper, demyelination of the optic nerves is a classic lesion. Occasionally, inflammation can extend into the optic nerve from panophthalmitis or from retrobulbar cellulitis (Figure 1.65).

(a)

(b)

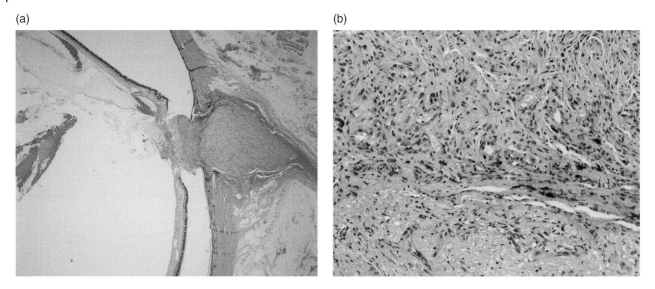

Figure 1.64 (a, b) Canine ocular gliovascular syndrome. The optic disk is gliotic and covered with a layer of fibrovascular tissue and glial cells that protrudes into the vitreous chamber.

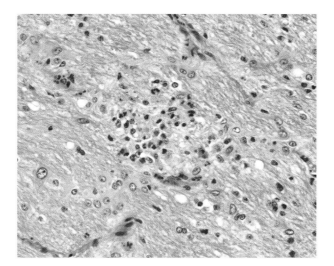

Figure 1.65 Optic neuritis due to aberrant migration of ascarid larvae. There is an infiltrate of eosinophils, macrophages and a few lymphocytes.

Granulomatous Meningoencephalitis

The idiopathic condition of canine granulomatous meningoencephalitis (GME) will occasionally extend into the optic nerves and meninges. This is characterized by an infiltrate of lymphocytes, macrophages, plasma cells, and occasionally a few pmns (Figure 1.66). The main differential diagnosis for optic nerve involvement would be lymphosarcoma.

Sclera

The sclera is the outer fibrous tunic of the eye, which is formed from periocular mesenchyme. It blends into the cornea at the limbus. The anterior portion of the sclera is covered by bulbar conjunctiva. The optic nerve exits the posterior of the globe through the lamina cribosa.

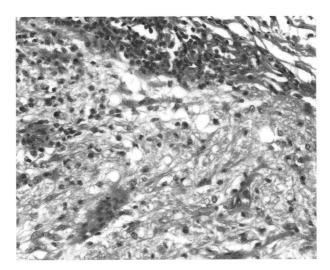

Figure 1.66   Optic neuritis due to due to granulomatous meningoencephalitis in a dog. There is an infiltrate of lymphocytes, plasma cells, and macrophages in the meninges and parenchyma of the nerve.

Developmental and Degenerative Scleral Disease

Scleral Ectasia

Occasionally, the sclera will be focally thinner than normal; this is **scleral ectasia**. It is typically associated with a defect in the closure of the optic fissure and coloboma of the choroid. Scleral ectasia and/or coloboma are commonly associated with choroidal hypoplasia and the **Collie eye anomaly** (Figure 1.67).

Inflammatory Disease of the Sclera

Lymphoplasmacytic Scleritis

Inflammation of the sclera, **scleritis**, does not usually occur alone; it most frequently accompanies uveitis or occasionally is a component of generalized eye inflammation (panophthalmitis) (Figure 1.68). Accumulation of lymphocytes and plasma cells around scleral vessels at the limbus or adjacent to the ciliary body is a common lesion that accompanies

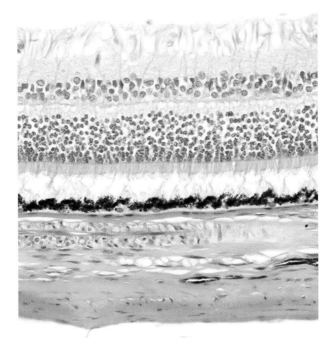

Figure 1.67   Scleral ectasia as a component of the Collie eye anomaly. The sclera is only about half of its normal thickness.

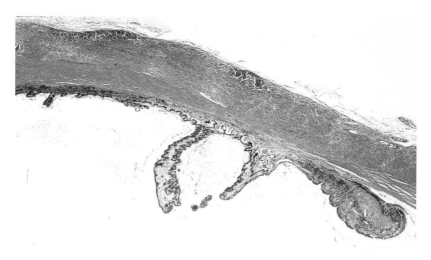

Figure 1.68 Lymphoplasmacytic scleritis. There is a perivascular to diffuse infiltrate of lymphocytes and plasma cells in the external surface of the sclera associated with chronic uveitis.

anterior uveitis. Occasionally, intraocular fungal diseases, such as blastomycosis, will extend through the wall of the eyeball and involve the sclera. Likewise, penetrating wounds into the eye that result in intraocular bacterial infection may also extend to involve the sclera.

Nodular Granulomatous Episcleritis and Necrotizing Scleritis

These are two apparently different syndromes that behave different clinically and have distinctive features and locations. Nodular granulomatous episcleritis (NGE) is more common and is composed of a mixture of macrophages, lymphocytes, plasma cells, and fibroblasts aligned in bundles and occurs in the bulbar conjunctiva at the limbus and may extend into the cornea; it also may occur on the membrana nictitans (Figure 1.69a). Necrotizing scleritis (NS) is a rare condition that contains foci of collagenolysis within the sclera along with a similar mix of inflammatory cells that may include granulomas. It is a more destructive lesion and may spread to involve the entire sclera and is frequently accompanied by lymphoplasmacytic uveitis (Figure 1.69b, c).

Eyelids, Conjunctiva and Retrobulbar Tissues

Developmental Disease of the Eyelids

The eyelids (palpebrae) are flaps of haired skin with a serous surface on the underside that is lined by palpebral conjunctiva. The edge of the eyelid contains a row of eyelashes (cilia) and associated sebaceous glands (Meibomian glands). The eyelids must meet properly to maintain an adequate tear film; eyelids that roll out (**ectropion)** or roll in (**entropion**) are unable to do this and result in eye irritation, especially the cornea. **Distichiasis** is the abnormal location of hairs along the eyelid margin; many times these will emerge from Meibomian gland openings. **Ectopic cilia** are frequently located on the conjunctival surface of the eyelid and cause irritation to the cornea.

Inflammatory Disease of the Eyelids

Granulomatous Blepharitis/Meibomian Adenitis

Blepharitis is inflammation of the eyelid. Inflammation of the Meibomian glands is Meibomian gland adenitis. Inflammation of these glands usually extends into the adjacent propria/submucosa causing blepharitis. **Granulomatous blepharitis** is the most common form of eyelid inflammation in the dog, and it is usually associated with leakage of secretion from the Meibomian glands. Granulomatous blepharitis typically forms a nodule along the lid margin, which is called a **chalazion** (Figure 1.70).

(a)

(b)

(c)

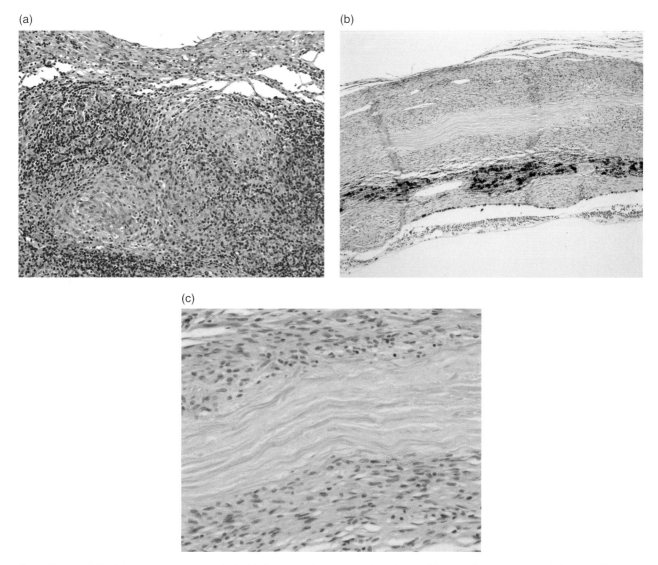

Figure 1.69   (a) Nodular granulomatous episcleritis in a dog. There is a multinodular infiltrate of lymphocytes and plasma cells associated with aggregates of macrophages in the external sclera. (b, c) Necrotizing scleritis in a dog. Also, there is lymphoplasmacytic uveitis and retinal atrophy.

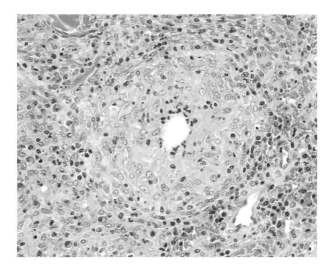

Figure 1.70   Granulomatous Meibomian blepharitis/adenitis (chalazion). This is a nodular sheet of epithelioid macrophages with a scattered infiltrate of lymphocytes, plasma cells and pmns centered on lipid material from a ruptured Meibomian gland.

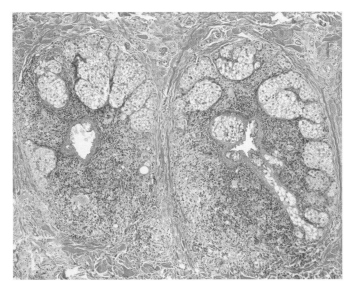

Figure 1.71   Marginal nodular Meibomian adenitis and blepharitis. This is granulomatous inflammation in multiple Meibomian glands along the eyelid margin.

Marginal Nodular Blepharitis/Meibomian Adenitis

This is an idiopathic disease recognized in dogs. It is characterized by multiple nodular foci of granulomatous inflammation involving multiple adjacent Meibomian glands along the eyelid margin (Figure 1.71).

Inflammatory Disease of the Conjunctiva, Membrana Nictitans, and Retrobulbar Tissues

The conjunctiva is located on the inner surface of the eyelid (palpebral conjunctiva) and the outer surface of the anterior portion of the sclera (bulbar conjunctiva). It is a thin layer of fibrovascular tissue that is covered with nonkeratinized stratified epithelium that varies from squamous to columnar. The membrana nictitans (third eyelid) is a specialized component of the conjunctiva, which is present at the medial canthus. In addition, to its serous mucosal surface, it contains a plate of cartilage, a lacrimal gland, and lymphoid tissue. In addition to the optic nerve and vessels that supply the eye, the retrobulbar tissue contains adipose tissue, extraocular muscles of the eye, and lacrimal gland.

Conjunctivitis

Conjunctivitis is inflammation of the conjunctiva. This is usually non-specific and due to irritation from foreign objects, dust, or chemicals. However, there are a few specific infectious agents that will produce conjunctivitis, such as *Chlamydophila felis* in cats. Inflammation of the membrana nictitans is a form of conjunctivitis.

Nodular Granulomatous Episcleritis/Conjunctivitis

This is inflammation of the bulbar conjunctiva and superficial sclera, which may extend into the cornea. The most common syndrome in dogs is **nodular granulomatous episcleritis** (Figure 1.72a, b). This is an idiopathic disease, which tends to begin at the lateral limbus and form indistinct nodular lesions. Occasionally NGE extends into the cornea and may occur on the membrana nictitans.

Periocular/Retrobulbar Cellulitis/Abscess

Inflammation may develop in the tissues (including salivary and lacrimal glands) behind or adjacent to the eye. This can be caused by a penetrating or migrating foreign object, but most of the time, the cause is not clear. Typically purulent exudate will accumulate in the retrobulbar tissue, sometimes forming an abscess. This will result in **exophthalmos** and occasionally, secondary ulcerative keratitis.

(a) (b)

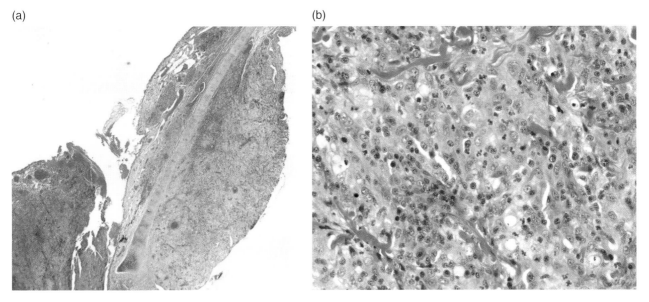

Figure 1.72 (a, b) Nodular granulomatous episcleritis/conjunctivitis on the membrana nictitans in a dog. There is a multinodular infiltrate of lymphocytes and plasma cells associated with aggregates of macrophages in the mucosa, extending down to the tarsal plate.

Neoplasia of the Eye and Periocular Tissues

Neoplasia of the Cornea

Primary neoplasia of the cornea is rare. Neoplasia within the cornea typically has invaded from a neoplasm that originates in the conjunctiva or anterior uvea. The most common primary neoplasm of the cornea is **squamous cell carcinoma** (Figure 1.73a, b). Although SCC can arise within the corneal epithelium, more commonly it originates in the adjacent conjunctiva and invades the cornea. **Squamous papilloma** also may occur (Figure 1.74a, b). **Uveal melanoma** may invade the cornea, tracking along Descemet's membrane, and **epibulbar melanoma** may invade into the cornea (Figure 1.75). There has been one case of a primary corneal melanoma with junctional activity reported in a horse. Also, there has been one case of a **primary corneal fibrosarcoma** in a cat, which was associated with a corneal ulcer and sequestrum (Figure 1.76a, b). **Hemangiosarcoma** has been reported to occur (Figure 1.77a, b).

(a) (b)

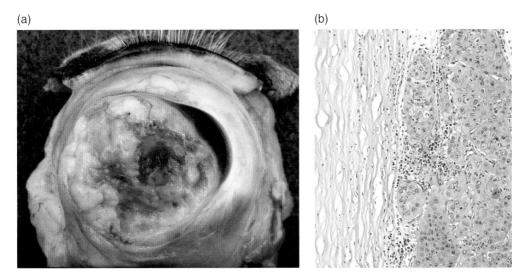

Figure 1.73 (a, b) Squamous cell carcinoma in the cornea of a horse.

(a) (b)

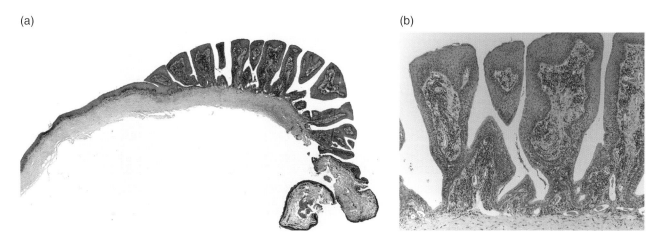

Figure 1.74 (a, b) Squamous papilloma on the corneal surface adjacent to the limbus.

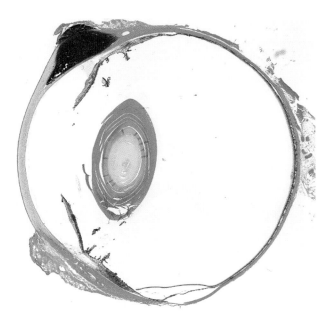

Figure 1.75 Canine epibulbar melanoma extending into the cornea.

(a) (b)

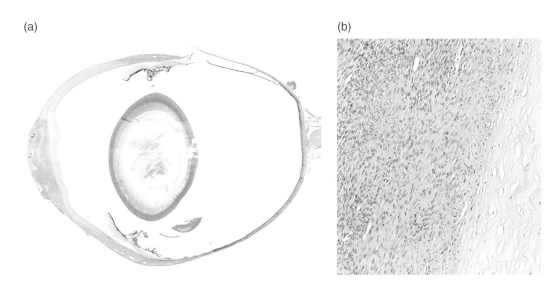

Figure 1.76 (a, b) Primary feline corneal fibrosarcoma.

(a)

(b)

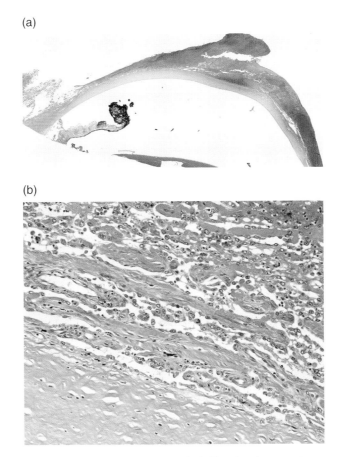

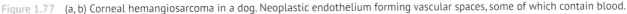

Figure 1.77   (a, b) Corneal hemangiosarcoma in a dog. Neoplastic endothelium forming vascular spaces, some of which contain blood.

Neoplasia of the Uvea

Intraocular Melanoma and Uveal Melanocytosis

Most intraocular melanomas originate in the anterior uvea. Uveal melanomas are very common in dogs, cats, and occasionally horses. **Canine uveal melanoma** is typically benign and originates in the iris or ciliary body; these typically are composed of heavily pigmented, round to spindle cells with a low mitotic index (Figure 1.78a, b). They may extend into the choroid and occasionally sclera; they can become fairly large and cause intraocular hemorrhage or secondary glaucoma. Intraocular melanoma in horses typically involves the anterior uvea and are benign. In cats, the typical melanocytic tumor is **diffuse iris melanoma**; these are considered to be malignant, and therefore may metastasize to other organs, although this is not very common. However, diffuse iris melanoma in cats will typically spread throughout the uvea and may obliterate much of the inner segments of the eye. Microscopically, the neoplastic cells can be quite pleomorphic and vary from well-differentiated round cells with a moderate amount of finely granular light brown pigment to very large round cells with one to several large nuclei with prominent nucleoli and minimal pigment (Figure 1.79a, b). Another condition that occurs primarily in Cairn Terriers is **uveal melanosis** (Figure 1.80). This condition is usually bilateral and characterized by progressive proliferation of heavily pigmented melanocytes in the anterior uvea that can extend along the scleral veins and exfoliate into the ciliary cleft and vitreous chamber. Uveal melanosis results in thickening of the affected iris and ciliary body and may be difficult to distinguish from a typical uveal melanoma. Also, it can cause secondary glaucoma.

Iridociliary Tumors

Ciliary body adenoma and adenocarcinoma are neoplasms derived from the neuroepithelium covering the ciliary body and/or the posterior surface of the iris. These are most common in the dog and are usually benign; even tumors that have cytological changes indicative of malignancy do not invade through the globe or metastasize. These are composed of cuboidal cells aligned in cords, tubules, or pseudotubules around vessels (Figure 1.81a–c). Iridociliary tumors frequently contain

(a)

(b)

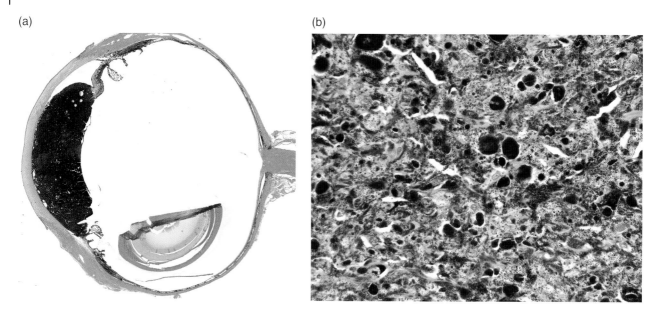

Figure 1.78 (a, b) Canine uveal melanoma. This uveal melanoma has developed within the iris and has formed anterior synechiae and partially closed the iridocorneal angle. The neoplastic melanocytes are large, round, heavily-pigmented cells. Also, the lens is luxated.

(a)

(b)

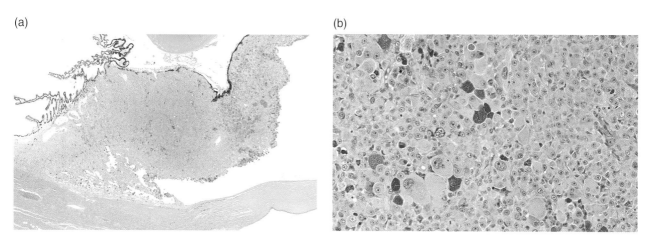

Figure 1.79 (a) Feline diffuse iris melanoma. This uveal melanoma has developed within the iris and has expanded into the ciliary body and closed the iridocorneal angle. (b) Marked anisocytosis and anisokaryosis with variable amounts of cytoplasmic pigmentation are common features.

basement membrane material surrounding lobules, foci of necrosis, are prone to hemorrhage and may stimulate the production of a PIFM.

Anterior Uveal Sarcoma of Blue-Eyed Dogs
This is an aggressive sarcoma that develops in the anterior uvea of dog breeds that typically have blue eyes, especially Siberian huskies (Figure 1.82a, b).

Intraocular Osteosarcoma
These are uncommon but occur, especially in the dog. These are aggressive neoplasms that obliterate all structures within the globe, so it is difficult to determine the specific intraocular site of origin. Their microscopic appearance is similar to osteosarcomas that occur in the appendicular skeleton (Figure 1.83a, b).

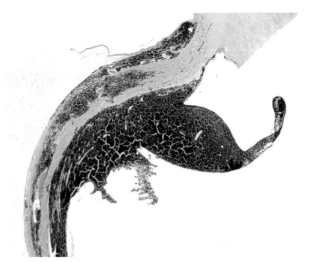

Figure 1.80 Uveal melanosis of Cairn Terriers. There is a diffuse infiltrate of large, heavily pigmented melanocytes and melanophages expanding the uvea and extending along scleral vessels.

(a)

(b)

(c)

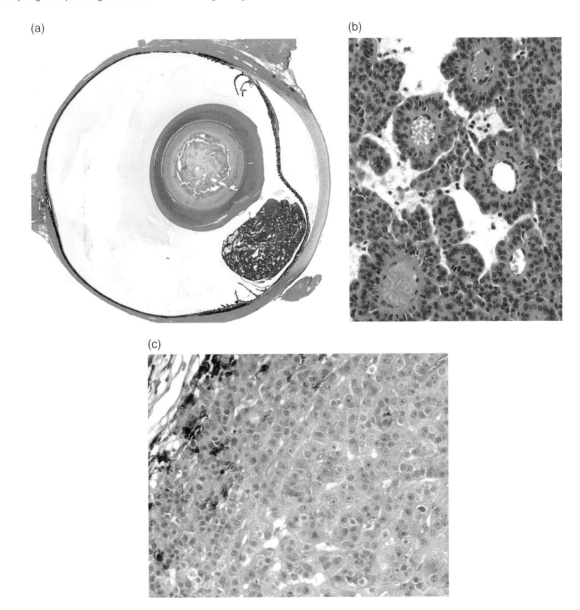

Figure 1.81 (a) Iridociliary tumor. These arise from the neuroepithelium covering the ciliary body and are typically a benign circumscribed mass. (b, c) These arise from the neuroepithelium covering the ciliary body and are composed of cells aligned in cords, tubules, or pseudotubules around vessels.

(a)

(b)

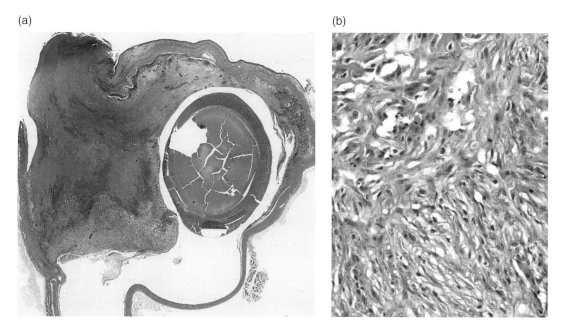

Figure 1.82   (a, b) Uveal sarcoma of blue-eyed dogs. This is an invasive poorly-differentiated sarcoma originating in the uvea.

(a)

(b)

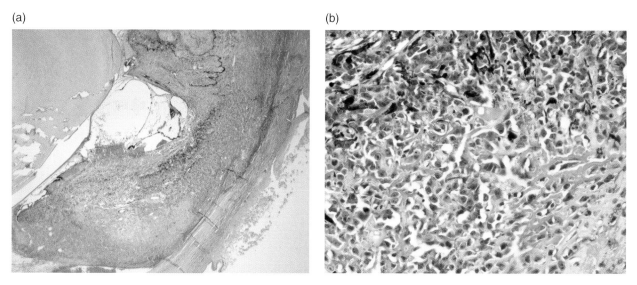

Figure 1.83   (a, b) Intraocular osteosarcoma. This is an invasive sarcoma that appears to originate in the uvea. It is composed of pyriform to polyhedral cells, some of which are surrounded by wisps of osteoid.

Intraocular Adenocarcinosarcoma (Malignant Mixed Tumor)

This is an uncommon malignant neoplasm that contains both neoplastic epithelial glandular tissue and mesenchymal tissue, which may include bone and/or cartilage (Figure 1.84).

Lymphoma

Ocular involvement is fairly common in lymphoma in most species. Usually, the uvea, including the choroid, is primarily infiltrated with neoplastic lymphocytes, which may efface the normal architecture, as in other tissues (Figure 1.85a–d). Ocular lymphoma may be a component of multicentric lymphoma, or it may apparently be limited to the eye. A form of lymphoma known as **presumed solitary ocular lymphoma (PSOL)** has been recognized in dogs and cats and may have a better prognosis than intraocular lymphoma that is a component of multicentric lymphoma. The immunophenotype of intraocular lymphoma can be B-cell, T-cell, or non-B/non-T cell.

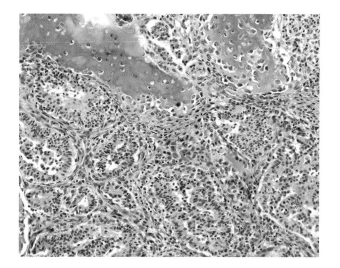

Figure 1.84 Intraocular adenocarcinosarcoma (malignant mixed tumor). This is an invasive neoplasm that appears to originate in the uvea. It is composed of cuboidal to columnar cells aligned in tubuloacinar structures along with polyhedral to spindle cells, some of which are surrounded by wisps of osteoid or bone.

(a)

(b)

(c)

(d)

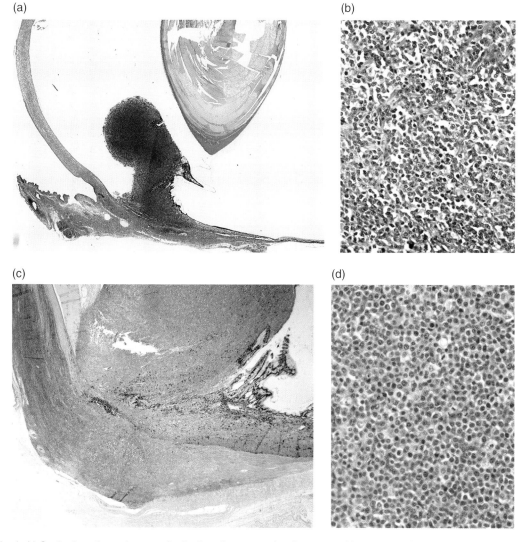

Figure 1.85 (a, b) Ocular lymphoma in a cat. Ocular lymphoma may involve any or all segments of the uvea. In this slide, an infiltrate of neoplastic lymphocytes has expanded and distorted the iris and ciliary body and has extended into the cornea and sclera. (c, d) Ocular lymphoma in a dog. Ocular lymphoma may be limited to the eye (presumed solitary ocular lymphoma), involving any or all segments of the uvea, or it may be a component of systemic lymphoma. In this slide, an infiltrate of neoplastic lymphocytes has expanded and distorted the iris and ciliary body and has extended into the cornea and sclera.

(a)

(b)

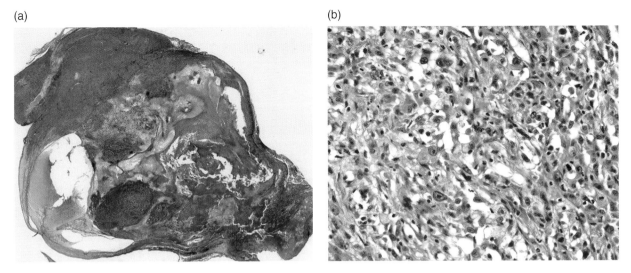

Figure 1.86 (a, b) Feline trauma-induced intraocular sarcoma. This is an invasive poorly-differentiated sarcoma that is presumed to originate from lens fiber epithelium following traumatic injury of the lens.

Neoplasia of the Lens

Trauma-Induced Intraocular Sarcoma of Cats

Trauma-induced intraocular sarcoma (TIIS) is a malignant neoplasm that is unique to cats. It occurs in an eye that has been severely traumatized, usually with a penetrating injury that has ruptured the lens capsule. It takes months to years to develop. It is thought to be due to neoplastic transformation of the lens epithelium, a step beyond fibrous metaplasia. Morphologically, TIIS can vary from a fibrosarcoma to osteosarcoma, and they frequently contain an infiltrate of lymphocytes and foci of necrosis. These typically invade circumferentially within the globe, obliterating all internal ocular components and can extend through the sclera into the periocular tissue (Figure 1.86a, b).

Neoplasia of the Retina

Primary neoplasia of the retina is extremely rare. Retinoblastoma and astrocytoma have been reported (Figure 1.87a–d).

Neoplasia of the Eyelids

Palpebral Melanocytoma and Malignant Melanoma

Melanomas and melanocytomas frequently occur on the eyelids as pedunculated or sessile masses, similar to other locations on the skin. These are typically benign, but many will have junctional activity. Neoplastic cells may vary from round with abundant pigment to spindle-shaped with little or no pigment (Figure 1.88a, b). Malignant melanoma of the eyelid in dogs is not common but microscopically resembles those of the oral cavity. These are invasive, rapidly growing neoplasms that frequently have satellite foci within the adjacent substantia propria and junctional activity (Figure 1.89a–c).

Squamous Cell Carcinoma

This is one of the most common neoplasms of the eyelids, third eyelid, and conjunctiva in dogs, cats, and horses. In draft horses, SCC is frequently multifocal and bilateral. Animals with little pigment in the eyelids are at increased risk due to the effect of ultraviolet radiation.

Squamous Papilloma

This is a common benign neoplasm that occurs on the eyelids of dogs. They may be caused by canine papillomavirus and are identical to those that occur in the skin and oral cavity.

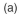

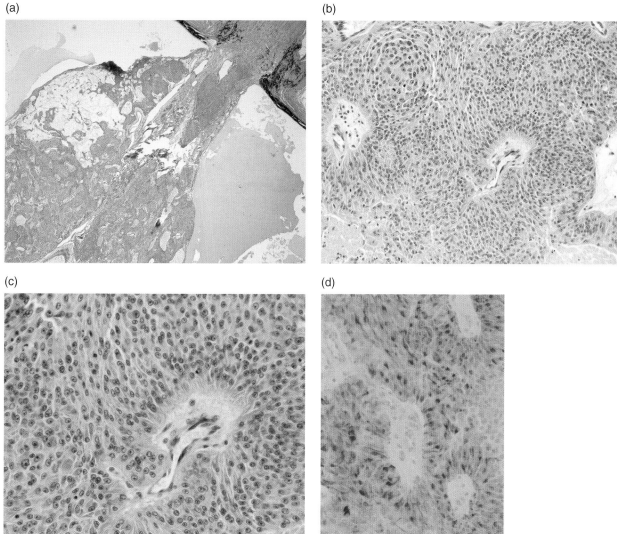

Figure 1.87   (a, b) Retinal astrocytoma. This is composed of polyhedral to spindle cells, some of which are aligned perpendicularly to the vessels. (c, d) These cells are immunoreactive for glial fibrillary acidic protein.

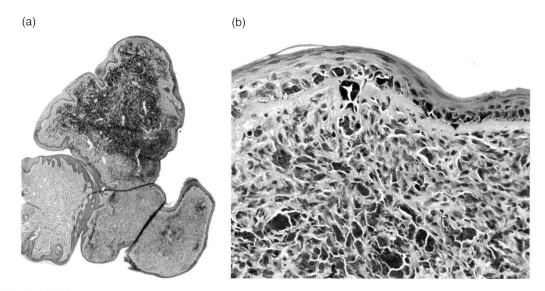

Figure 1.88   (a, b) Melanoma on the eyelid. Heavily pigmented cells are typical of melanoma in this location. Note the pigmented neoplastic cells within the epidermis; this is junctional activity.

(a)

(b)

(c)

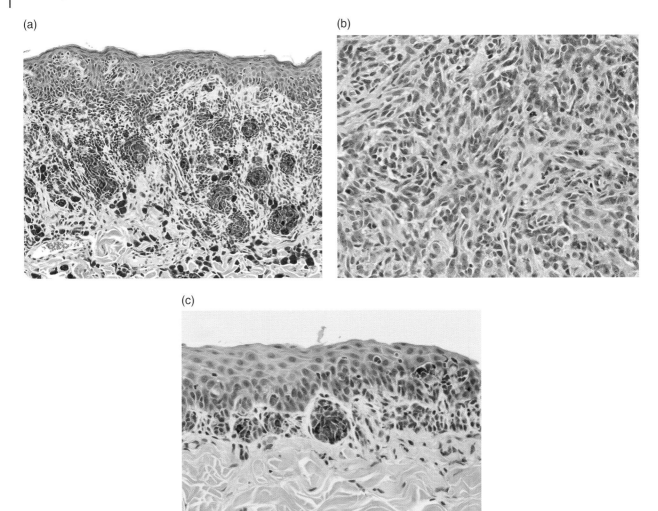

Figure 1.89 (a) Malignant melanoma on the eyelid. Heavily pigmented round cells along with poorly-pigmented spindle cells. Note the pigmented neoplastic cells within the epidermis (junctional activity). (b) Poorly-pigmented spindle cells with high mitotic index. (c) Aggregates of pigmented neoplastic cells within the epidermis (junctional activity).

Meibomian Gland Tumors

Meibomian gland tumors are extremely common in old dogs and less so in cats; they resemble sebaceous tumors that commonly occur in the skin. **Focal Meibomian hyperplasia** is typically a small mass that still retains some degree of gland architecture (Figure 1.90). **Meibomian adenoma** is typically a pedunculated mass on the eyelid margin composed of multiple lobules of well-differentiated sebaceous glands surrounding a duct lined by stratified squamous epithelium (Figure 1.91a, b). **Meibomian epithelioma** is less differentiated and is predominantly composed of proliferative basal reserve cells with scattered sebocytes; these are considered to be a premalignant lesion (Figure 1.92). Occasionally, **Meibomian adenocarcinoma** occurs. It is common for any of these Meibomian tumors to be ulcerated and partially surrounded by granulomatous to pyogranulomatous exudate (chalazion) secondary to trauma.

Neoplasia of the Conjunctiva and Membrana Nictitans

Squamous Cell Carcinoma

Squamous cell carcinoma is a serious disease of the conjunctiva and typically occurs on the third eyelid and bulbar conjunctiva in white-face horses, dogs, and cats (Figure 1.93a, b).

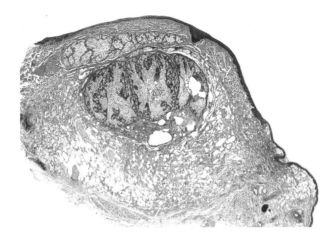

Figure 1.90   Meibomian gland hyperplasia surrounded by granulomatous inflammation.

(a)   (b)

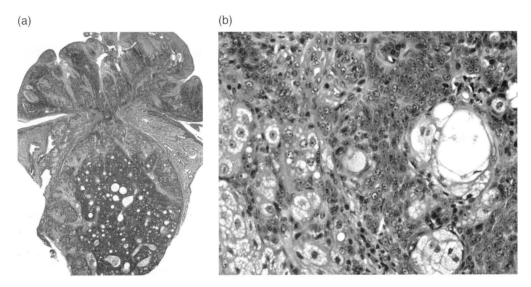

Figure 1.91   (a, b) Meibomian gland adenoma. These are nodular or papillomatous masses composed of lobules of well-differentiated sebocytes and a moderate number of spindle-shaped basal cells along with small ductular structures.

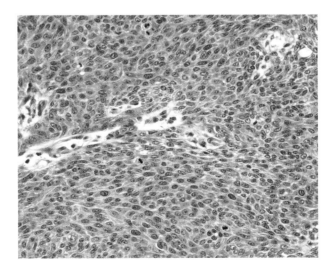

Figure 1.92   Meibomian gland epithelioma. These are composed primarily of spindle-shaped basal cells and a few scattered sebocytes. The mitotic index is typically high.

(a)   (b)

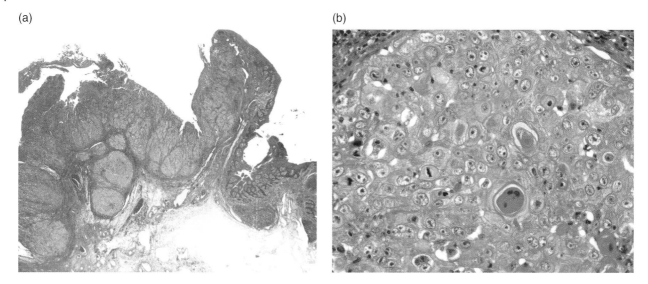

Figure 1.93 (a) Squamous cell carcinoma on the third eyelid. (b) Neoplastic cells are round to polygonal, have a large round to oval nucleus, one to two prominent nucleoli, abundant eosinophilic cytoplasm, and prominent desmosomes. Occasional cells are keratinized.

(a)   (b)

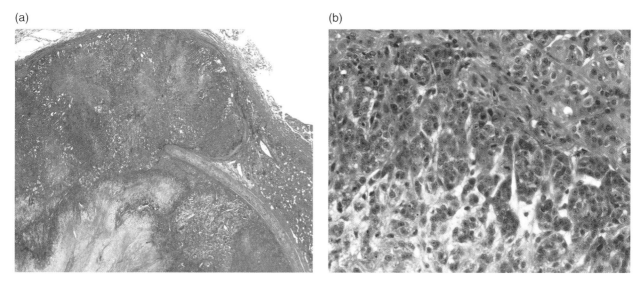

Figure 1.94 (a, b) Adenocarcinoma of the gland of the third eyelid. Neoplastic cells are cuboidal and are aligned in clusters or crude tubuloacinar structures.

Adenocarcinoma of Gland of Third Eyelid (Membrana Nictitans)

These are rare neoplasms in all species but are most common in old dogs. Microscopically, they are locally invasive and are composed of cells that are cuboidal and aligned in clusters or crude tubuloacinar structures (Figure 1.94a, b).

Epibulbar Melanoma

Melanomas also occur on the surface of the globe at the limbus in dogs. These are called limbal or **epibulbar melanomas**; they are considered to be benign.

Neoplasia of Retrobulbar Tissues

Retrobulbar Meningioma

Occasionally, a meningioma will develop in the meninges surrounding the optic nerve in dogs. These have a similar microscopic appearance to meningiomas in the CNS that are composed of spindle to polyhedral cells aligned in small sheets or clusters that frequently have a swirled pattern (Figure 1.95a–c). However, a distinctive feature that is common in

(a)

(b)

(c)

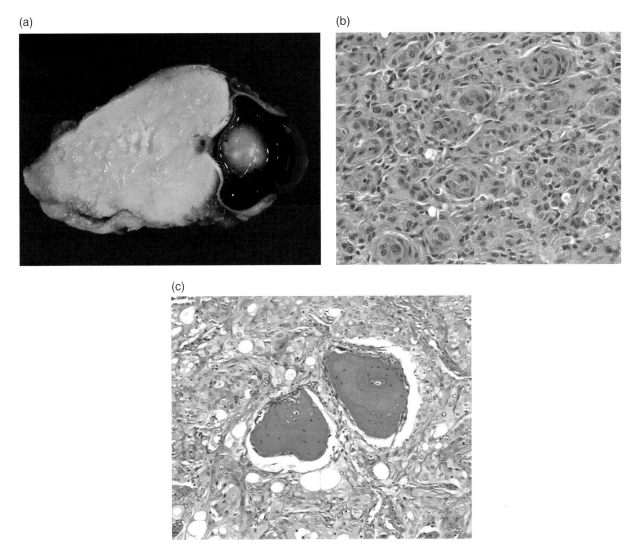

Figure 1.95   (a, b) Canine retrobulbar meningioma. (c) In addition to clusters or swirls of neoplastic spindle to polyhedral cells, these neoplasms commonly contain foci of metaplastic bone and cartilage.

retrobulbar meningiomas is foci of metaplastic bone and cartilage. Biologically, these neoplasms are generally benign, but they will surround the optic nerve and compress the globe frequently producing exophthalmos and atrophy of the optic nerve.

Retrobulbar Peripheral Nerve Sheath Tumor
Occasionally these arise from nerves within the orbit, branches of cranial nerves III, IV, and VI. They resemble peripheral nerve sheath tumors of the limbs and are characterized by interlacing, palisading, and swirling bundles of spindle cells (Figure 1.96).

Lymphoma
Multicentric lymphoma may develop in the retrobulbar tissues and surround and invade into the optic nerve.

Adenoma/Adenocarcinoma of Lacrimal Gland or Zygomatic Salivary Gland
There are several possible glandular neoplasms that occur in the retrobulbar/periocular tissues, but these are difficult to distinguish from each other. Adenomas of the lacrimal gland and zygomatic salivary gland have a very similar microscopic appearance and are mainly distinguished based on their location. These are circumscribed neoplasms composed of cuboidal to columnar epithelium aligned in multiple acinar structures (Figure 1.97). Adenocarcinoma of the lacrimal or zygomatic gland is composed of invasive cuboidal to columnar epithelium aligned in multiple crude acinar structures separated by immature fibrous tissue (desmoplastic response) (Figure 1.98).

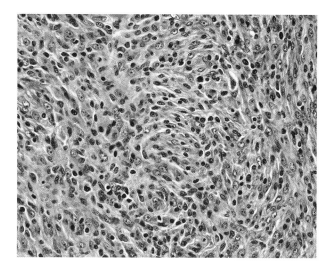

Figure 1.96   Retrobulbar nerve sheath tumor. Interlacing, palisading, and swirling bundles of spindle cells are characteristic. These may also contain an infiltrate of lymphocytes.

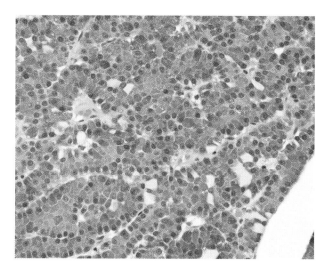

Figure 1.97   Lacrimal gland adenoma. This is composed of cuboidal to columnar epithelium aligned in multiple acinar structures.

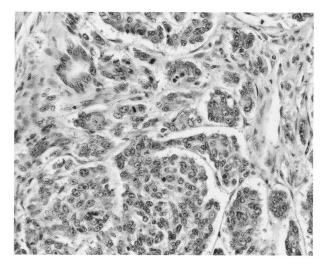

Figure 1.98   Lacrimal gland adenocarcinoma. This is composed of invasive cuboidal to columnar epithelium aligned in multiple crude acinar structures separated by immature fibrous tissue.

(a) (b)

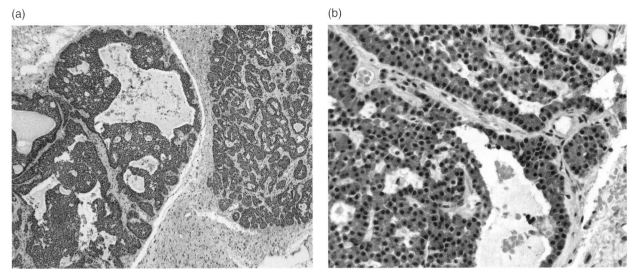

Figure 1.99   (a, b) Canine orbital lobular adenoma. This is composed of multiple lobules of well-differentiated cuboidal to columnar epithelium aligned in acini. The lobules are separated by loose fibrovascular tissue that makes the mass very friable and poorly demarcated.

Canine Orbital Lobular Adenoma

This is also a benign neoplasm that occurs in the retrobulbar tissues. It is composed of multiple lobules of well-differentiated cuboidal to columnar epithelium aligned in acini. The lobules are separated by loose fibrovascular tissue that makes the mass very friable and poorly demarcated; this is the main distinguishing feature of this neoplasm (Figure 1.99a, b).

References and Additional Readings

Komaromy, A.M., Abrams, K.L., Heckenlively, J.R. et al. (2016). Sudden acquired retinal degeneration syndrome (SARDS) – a review and proposed strategies toward a better understanding of pathogenesis, early diagnosis, and therapy. *Vet. Ophthalmol.* 19 (4): 319–331.

Beamer, G., Reilly, C.M., and Pizzirani, S. (2015). Microscopic lesions in canine eyes with primary glaucoma. *Vet. Clin. North Am. Small Anim. Pract.* 45 (6): 1213–1233. https://doi.org/10.1016/j.cvsm.2015.07.001.

Cooper, A.E., Ahonen, S., Rowlan, J.S. et al. (2014). A novel form of progressive retinal atrophy in Swedish vallhund dogs. *PLoS One* 9 (9): e106610. https://doi.org/10.1371/journal.pone.0106610. Erratum in: PLoS One 2015; 10(2): e0118128. PMID: 25198798; PMCID: PMC4157785.

Dean, E. and Meunier, V. (2013). Feline eosinophilic keratoconjunctivitis: a retrospective study of 45 cases (56 eyes). *J. Feline Med. Surg.* 15 (8): 661–666. https://doi.org/10.1177/1098612X12472181.

Deehr, A.J. and Dubielzig, R.R. (1998). A histopathological study of iridociliary cysts and glaucoma in Golden Retrievers. *Vet. Ophthalmol.* 1 (2–3): 153–158. https://doi.org/10.1046/j.1463-5224.1998.00018.x.

Denk, N., Sandmeyer, L.S., Lim, C.C. et al. (2012). A retrospective study of the clinical, histological, and immunohistochemical manifestations of 5 dogs originally diagnosed histologically as necrotizing scleritis. *Vet. Ophthalmol.* 15 (2): 102–109. https://doi.org/10.1111/j.1463-5224.2011.00948.x.

Gelatt, K.N., van der Woerdt, A., Ketring, K.L. et al. (2001). Enrofloxacin associated retinal degeneration in cats. *Vet. Ophthalmol.* 4 (2): 99–106.

Headrick, J.F., Bentley, E., and Dubielzig, R.R. (2004). Canine lobular orbital adenoma: a report of 15 cases with distinctive features. *Vet. Ophthalmol.* 7 (1): 47–51. https://doi.org/10.1111/j.1463-5224.2004.00323.x.

Grahn, B., Peiffer, R., and Wilcock, B. (2019). *Histologic Basis of Ocular Disease in Animals*. Wiley Blackwell.

Jost, H.E., Townsend, W.M., Moore, G.E., and Liang, S. (2020). Golden retriever pigmentary uveitis: vision loss, risk factors for glaucoma, and effect of treatment on disease progression. *Vet. Ophthalmol.* 23 (6): 1001–1008. https://doi.org/10.1111/vop.12841.

Maxie, M.G. (ed.) (2016). Chapter 5 – special senses. In: *Jubb, Kennedy and Palmer's Pathology of Domestic Animals*, 6e, vol. 1, 407–488. Brian Wilcock.

Lanza, M.R., Musciano, A.R., Dubielzig, R.D., and Durham, A.C. (2018). Clinical and pathological classification of canine intraocular lymphoma. *Vet. Ophthalmol.* 21 (2): 167–173.

Petersen-Jones, S.M., Mentzer, A.L., Dubielzig, R.R. et al. (2008). Ocular melanosis in the Cairn Terrier: histopathological description of the condition, and immunohistological and ultrastructural characterization of the characteristic pigment-laden cells. *Vet. Ophthalmol.* 11 (4): 260–268. https://doi.org/10.1111/j.1463-5224.2008.00640.x.

Sebbag, L., Riggs, A., and Carnevale, J. (2020). Oculo-skeletal dysplasia in five Labrador Retrievers. *Vet. Ophthalmol.* 23 (2): 386–393. https://doi.org/10.1111/vop.12715.

Treadwell, A., Naranjo, C., Blocker, T. et al. (2015). Clinical and histological characteristics of canine ocular gliovascular syndrome. *Vet. Ophthalmol.* 18 (5): 371–380. https://doi.org/10.1111/vop.12209.

Meuten, D. (ed.) Chapter 20 – tumors of the eye. In: *Tumors in Domestic Animals*, 5e, 892–922. Richard Dubielzig.

Gelatt, K. (ed.) (2007). *Veterinary Ophthalmology*, 4e. Blackwell Publishing.

Zarfoss, M.K., Tusler, C.A., Kass, P.H. et al. (2018). Clinical findings and outcomes for dogs with uveodermatologic syndrome. *J. Am. Vet. Med. Assoc.* 252 (10): 1263–1271. https://doi.org/10.2460/javma.252.10.1263.

Zeiss, C.J., Johnson, E.M., and Dubielzig, R.R. (2003). Feline intraocular tumors may arise from transformation of lens epithelium. *Vet. Pathol.* 40 (4): 355–362. https://doi.org/10.1354/vp.40-4-355.

2

Pathology of the Bones and Joints

Joseph S. Haynes

Department of Veterinary Pathology, Iowa State University, Ames, IA, USA

Introduction

Surgical specimens from the bones and joints are a fairly common submission for evaluation. However, with the exception of the amputated limb or digit that contains a skeletal mass, the specimens are frequently small and usually do not encompass the entire lesion. In fact, small specimens may not contain the primary lesion at all, which can lead to misdiagnosis. There are several reasons for this. First of all, skeletal tissue can be technically difficult to biopsy. Second, because bone has a limited range of responses to injury, very different primary lesions frequently incite the same secondary lesions, and a single small specimen may miss the primary lesion. An example of this would be osteosarcoma compared to a healing fracture or chronic osteomyelitis – all produce an osseous mass and all incite a substantial amount of proliferative new bone on the periosteal surface, but if the specimens do not contain neoplastic tissue from the osteosarcoma or exudate from the osteomyelitis, then these specimens could all have the same microscopic appearance. There are two factors that can help limit misdiagnoses of small biopsy specimens: 1. an accurate signalment and clinical history, including species, breed, age, sex, and location of the lesion, and 2. an accurate radiographic evaluation. This combination of signalment/history, radiographic appearance, and microscopic evaluation will provide the best chance for an accurate diagnosis.

Specimen Preparation, Fixation, and Demineralization

Osseous tissue is hard, and because of that, it requires special preparation. If the specimens are only a few millimeters thick, they can be directly immersed in 10% neutral buffered formalin for fixation. However, if the specimen is a centimeter or more in thickness, or if it is an entire lesion in a bone or joint from an amputated limb, then it will need to be dissected free of overlying soft tissue and sectioned with a saw into pieces 5 mm or so in thickness; cutting pieces thinner than this will frequently produce artifacts in the specimen. After cutting with a saw, these pieces should be gently rinsed in running water to remove any bits of "bone sawdust" adhered to the surface before they are immersed in formalin. Once the specimens have fixed, then they will usually need to be demineralized prior to sectioning with a razor blade. Demineralization is usually performed with a solution of formic acid or occasionally, EDTA. Prolonged demineralization will adversely affect the quality of subsequent staining, typically making the sections hypereosinophilic; so the shorter the duration of demineralization, the better. Once the specimen is demineralized, then it is cut to size with a razor blade and loaded into cassettes for processing. Specimens that were cut with a saw should be split down the center with a razor blade to produce a surface opposite the sawn surface from which microtome sections should be cut; this eliminates the artifactual incorporation of bone sawdust into the final microscopic slides.

Bone Structure and Physiology

A detailed review of bone and joint structure and physiology is beyond the scope of this book. What follows is a basic overview of bone and joint structure and physiology intended to set the tone for understanding the various reactions to injury that occur in osseous tissues. Those seeking a more detailed review are referred to the additional readings listed at the end of this chapter.

The skeleton is the hard scaffold of the body, yet it is living tissue. Bone is in a dynamic state capable of growth, modeling, remodeling, and repair. Modeling is involved with the initial sculpting of bones and is influenced by the distribution of skeletal load. Remodeling is the mechanism of continually renewing bone to accommodate redistribution of load on the skeleton; it occurs throughout the life of the animal and is composed of coordinated removal and production of bone.

Bone is composed of cells, extracellular matrix, mineral salts, and a variety of embedded molecules that help regulate bone growth and function. Osteoblasts are responsible for the synthesis of the premineralized bone matrix, osteoid. It is composed mostly of type I collagen and is responsible for the tensile strength of bone. Osteoblasts are cuboidal to columnar cells that are aligned along osteoid seams. Osteoblasts become bone-lining cells when they are not producing osteoid and osteocytes when they are incorporated into the bone matrix they have produced. Osteocytes reside is lacunae and have long cytoplasmic processes that extend through bone canaliculi. Osteocytes and bone-lining cells have receptors for parathyroid hormone (PTH) and are important in the minute-to-minute regulation of serum calcium concentration. Because they have PTH receptors and osteoclasts do not, they direct the formation and activity of osteoclasts in response to increased PTH (Figure 2.1). In addition, osteoblasts and osteocytes produce molecules and secrete them into the organic matrix, such as osteocalcin (aids in mineralization), bone morphogenetic proteins (a family of growth factors that stimulate bone growth), various cytokines, adhesion molecules, and enzymes, that help regulate the growth and function of bone. Deposition of osteoid occurs several days prior to mineralization. Mineral is first added to the organic matrix as amorphous calcium phosphate but is subsequently converted to a more stable, crystalline form of calcium phosphate, hydroxyapatite; mineral provides hardness and rigidity to bone, as well as a storage site for calcium and phosphorus. Osteoclasts are large multinucleated cells derived from hematopoietic stem cells that are responsible for the resorption of bone and calcified cartilage. They are important for modeling and remodeling of bone and are formed in response to M-CSF, RANK ligand, tumor necrosis factor (TNF), and/or IL1. These molecules are produced by osteoblasts, osteocytes, hypertrophic chondrocytes, and T-cells, and along with PTH, basically control osteoclast activity. Osteoclasts are either located individually in Howship's lacunae along the surface of a bone or in groups within Haversian canals known as cutting cones (Figure 2.2). Osteoclasis is the removal of bone by osteoclasts; it is a surface reaction that is due to the dissolution of minerals by acid followed by digestion of the organic matrix by enzymes. Removal of bone during remodeling is due to osteoclasis and proceeds at a more rapid rate in growing animals.

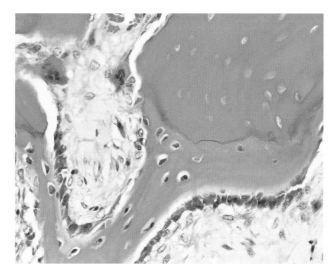

Figure 2.1   Osteoblasts lining trabecular bone laid down onto necrotic bone.

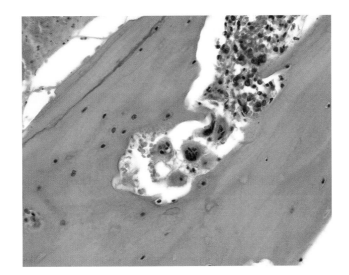

Figure 2.2   A cutting cone of osteoclasts within a Haversian canal.

Development of Bone and Cartilage

Bone develops via two main mechanisms: endochondral ossification and intramembranous ossification. Endochondral ossification involves calcification of a cartilaginous model with subsequent resorption and replacement by bone. Endochondral ossification occurs in developing long bones with primary and secondary centers of ossification. Bones formed via endochondral ossification have several anatomical zones. The diaphysis is the central portion of the bone and it contains the primary center of ossification. The epiphysis is at the end of a bone; it contains a secondary center of ossification and it has an articular surface covered with articular hyaline cartilage. The junction between the articular cartilage and the subchondral bone in the epiphysis is the articular–epiphyseal complex (AE complex); endochondral ossification occurs here, which is necessary for the articular surface to acquire its appropriate conformation. The physis is the zone of growth cartilage that is the remnant of the cartilage model and persists until the bone reaches maturity. It is a polarized structure that is bordered by a bone-formative surface, the metaphysis that is located on the diaphyseal side. There is a metaphysis at each end of the diaphysis and this is where the primary spongiosa (newest trabecular bone) is located. All bones are covered by a periosteum, which is composed of a tough outer fibrous layer that provides support and serves as an attachment site for muscle, tendons and ligaments, and an inner cambium layer that supplies blood to the cortical bone and also contains stem cells that will produce new bone in response to periosteal injury.

Intramembranous ossification predominates in the skull and facial bones. During intramembranous ossification, there is production of interweaving bundles of coarse collagen fibrils that are termed "woven bone"; this woven bone contains osteoblasts and osteocytes but is not as orderly as bone formed by endochondral ossification (Figure 2.3a, b). Woven bone is temporary; it is produced relatively quickly but is later modeled and remodeled into lamellar bone. Appositional bone growth is essentially intramembranous ossification that occurs along the shafts of long bones and increases long bone diameter.

Bone is organized into several different patterns, depending upon its location and function. These are cortical bone, trabecular bone, lamellar bone, woven bone and osteons. Cortical bone is the densest pattern and is composed of lamellar bone organized into multiple osteons. Osteons have a central Haversian canal that is surrounded by concentric layers of lamellar bone. The Haversian canal contains vessels, nerves, osteoblasts and osteoclasts. Trabecular bone is composed of interconnecting bands of bone that span the medullary cavity of bones and form the subchondral bone plates beneath articular cartilage. It is composed of lamellar bone but does not typically contain osteons.

Cartilage is an important component of the developing, immature and mature skeleton. In the developing skeleton, it forms the cartilage models for endochondral ossification; remnants of these cartilage models persist in the immature skeleton as growth plates or physes. Cartilage is produced by chondroblasts in much the same way as osteoblasts produce bone. Chondrocytes are the cells that are located within lacunae in the cartilaginous matrix. These cells have different shapes depending upon their state of differentiation and function. The matrix of cartilage involved in endochondral ossification is composed of proteoglycan aggregates, type X collagen and abundant water. In the mature skeleton, cartilage is only present

(a)

(b)

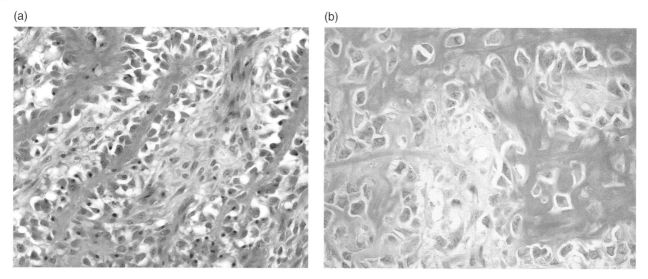

Figure 2.3   (a, b) Woven bone within an area of hyperostosis.

on articular surfaces and it has a somewhat different structure, containing types II and IX collagen that are structural. Articular cartilage lacks a blood supply and is nourished by the synovial fluid. The deepest layer of articular cartilage is characterized by a distinct layer of mineralized matrix that is attached to the subchondral bone plate by collagen fibers. The proteoglycan aggregates are large, hydrophilic and are composed of a hyaluronic acid backbone and core protein side chains that are decorated with keratan sulfate and chondroitin sulfate.

Basic Reactions of Bone to Injury

Bone has a limited set of reactions to injury that include hypoplastic/dysplastic growth, bone loss, excessive bone production, necrosis, inflammation, and neoplasia. Many bone lesions consist of various combinations of these reactions. So a discussion of these reactions as they occur in bone is an important prelude to a discussion of specific bone diseases.

Hypoplastic/Dysplastic Bone Growth

Osseous hypoplasia can be the result of a genetic defect, as occurs in osteogenesis imperfecta, or may be acquired due to nutritional abnormalities, toxicity, or even systemic illness (Figure 2.4). This may cause an abnormality of endochondral ossification, and thus, the primary lesion is in the cartilage of the physes and/or articular–epiphyseal complex. When

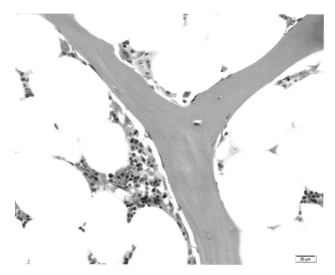

Figure 2.4   This is osseous hypoplasia due to osteogenesis imperfect in a dog.

general nutrient deficiency occurs or when prolonged anorexia develops in a young animal, endochondral ossification may stop, and a thin plate of bone will develop along the metaphyseal side of the growth plate; this is a **growth arrest line**. When the cause is alleviated, endochondral ossification may begin again, but the growth arrest line of bone will persist until it is remodeled. A **growth retardation lattice** is a different abnormality that is caused by some agent (toxic or infectious) that kills osteoclasts in the primary spongiosa; this results in the failure of modeling of the small bone trabeculae of the primary spongiosa into larger trabeculae of the medulla.

Much of the time, **dysplastic bone growth** is caused by a genetic defect, as in chondrodysplastic dwarfism, but it may also be caused by acquired injury to one or more of the physes or A–E complexes. Dysplastic bone growth usually manifests grossly as shortened bones with angular deformities. Microscopic changes may be subtle, but when present, may include disorganization and thickening of the physes, inappropriate or diminished mineralization of the physes, or premature closure of the physes.

Loss of Bone

Loss of bone may be either diffuse or localized. Diffuse bone loss is usually called **osteoporosis**, while localized bone loss is usually called **osteolysis**. **Osteoporosis** is basically atrophy of bone. The bone that is present is normal, but there is just too little of it. It occurs when bone resorption is greater than bone formation. Many conditions can cause this including disuse, uncomplicated calcium deficiency, dietary protein deficiency, estrogen deficiency (in postmenopausal women), copper deficiency, and hypovitaminosis A and/or C. It often manifests clinically as multiple pathologic fractures, especially of the lumbar spine, pelvis, and femurs. **Focal or multifocal osteolysis** is the result of local intense osteoclasis, usually in response to inflammation or neoplasia (Figure 2.5). Focal osteolysis is especially common with metastatic neoplasms in bone.

Excessive Production of Bone

The general term for excessive production of bone is **hyperostosis** (Figure 2.6). This is basically bone hypertrophy and hyperplasia secondary to injury. It is a common chronic reaction to trauma, infection, neoplasia, and a few nutritional abnormalities, such as hypervitaminosis A or D. Also, there are several idiopathic conditions that have hyperostosis as a characteristic lesion, including craniomandibular osteopathy. Usually, the new bone that is produced is woven bone on the periosteal surface. However, new bone may be produced on the endosteal surface, where it is more likely to be lamellar bone. The orientation of initial bone deposition by the periosteum has a characteristic pattern of spicules oriented perpendicular to the cortical surface; this same pattern occurs regardless of the cause. Over time, the woven bone will be remodeled into lamellar bone. The general term for a focal area of hyperostosis is **exostosis**; the specific term for one that occurs at the attachment site of the joint capsule is **periarticular osteophyte**, and one that occurs at the attachment site of a tendon or ligament is **enthesophyte**. Usually, periarticular osteophytes will also contain cartilage (Figure 2.7).

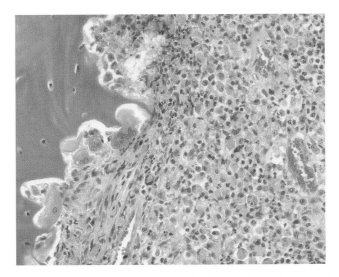

Figure 2.5 This is focal osteolysis associated with chronic osteomyelitis. Note the layer of osteoclasts within Howship's lacunae along the scalloped edge of trabecular bone.

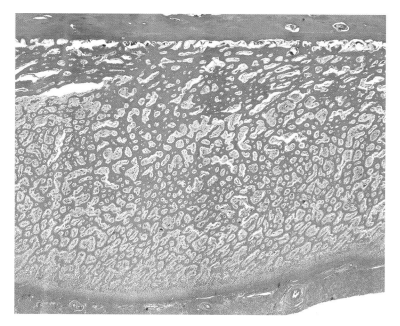

Figure 2.6   This is hyperostosis on the cortical surface of a bone. The newest bone spicules are adjacent to the periosteum, and their orientation is generally perpendicular to the cortical surface.

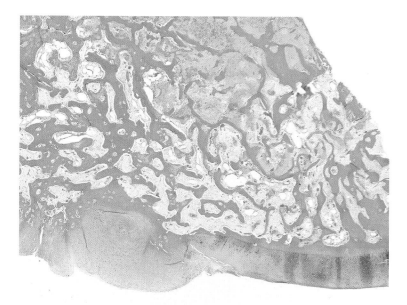

Figure 2.7   This is a periarticular osteophyte expanding the left edge of the articular cartilage.

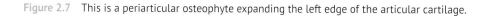

Osteonecrosis

Osteonecrosis occurs under a variety of circumstances, but it is most commonly due to ischemia. Interruption of arterial supply or venous drainage will lead to ischemia. Bone necrosis is usually only recognized clinically when it involves bone that is adjacent to an articular surface or when it is separated from the parent bone in the form of a **sequestrum** (Figure 2.8). There is typically some degree of necrosis in the bone on either side of a fracture. Grossly, necrotic bone may be chalky and usually contains pale marrow. Microscopically, the lacunae are empty, there are no osteoblasts lining the trabeculae, and the marrow is necrotic (Figure 2.9). Later, as a healing response, new bone is produced upon the surface of the necrotic bone, and the marrow is replaced by fibrous tissue (Figure 2.10).

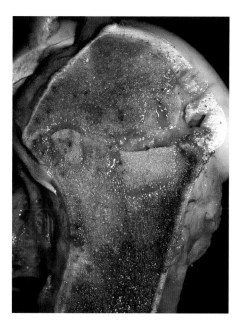

Figure 2.8   This is chronic purulent osteomyelitis with several sequestra.

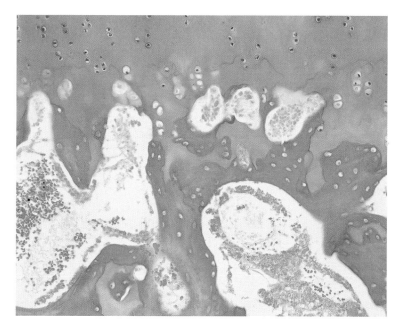

Figure 2.9   This is osteonecrosis of the femoral head. The lacunae in the necrotic subchondral bone are either empty or contain remnants of necrotic osteocytes. Also note that the tissue in the medullary spaces is necrotic.

Inflammation of Bone

Inflammation of a bone is **osteitis**; if the marrow is also inflamed (which is almost always the case), the condition is **osteomyelitis**. **Periosteitis** is inflammation of the periosteum. Acute inflammation of bone is characterized by accumulation of fibrinous to purulent exudate, and frequently, osteonecrosis. However, by the time osteomyelitis is recognized, it has usually progressed to a chronic phase, characterized by both osteoblastic and osteoclastic activity in varying degrees. Osteitis occurs not only with infection but also in response to tissue damage from other causes such as trauma or foreign bodies. In infectious osteomyelitis, bacteria are more likely to play an important role if there is venous thrombosis or

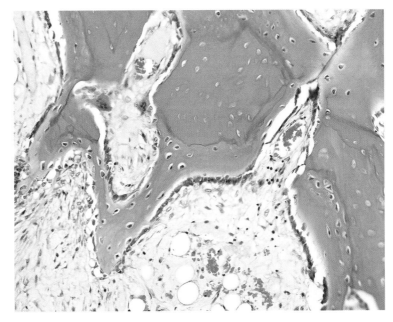

Figure 2.10   Bone infarct. The necrotic bone acts as a scaffold for new bone production. Note the robust row of osteoblasts lining the surface of the new bone. Also, the marrow has been replaced by loose fibrovascular tissue.

vascular occlusion allowing bacteria to grow and colonize. The three routes of infection are through the bloodstream (hematogenous), a penetrating wound, or direct extension from an infection in the adjacent soft tissue. Hematogenous bacterial infections tend to occur in young animals and usually develop at the metaphysis or A/E complex. Bacteria preferentially localize at the ends of the metaphyseal capillaries because these capillaries have endothelial fenestrations that allow bacteria to exit. In addition, the local defense mechanism is weak and easily overwhelmed because the local phagocytes seem to have difficulty in killing bacteria.

Suppurative osteomyelitis is perhaps the most common form of osteomyelitis, and it is the typical response of bone to infection by most types of bacteria. Bacterial products, ischemia and neutrophil enzymes cause necrosis of marrow and often, trabecular bone (Figure 2.11). Persistent, progressive infections are common and cause **chronic suppurative**

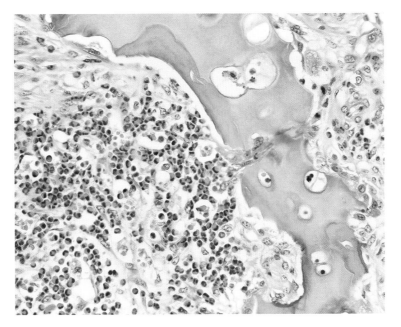

Figure 2.11   Suppurative osteomyelitis.

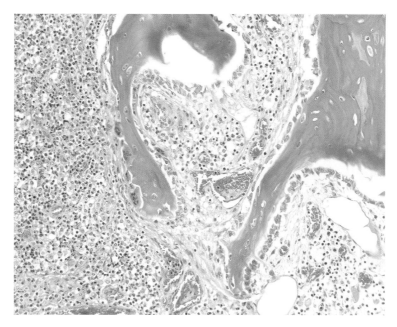

Figure 2.12   This is chronic suppurative osteomyelitis with osteolysis.

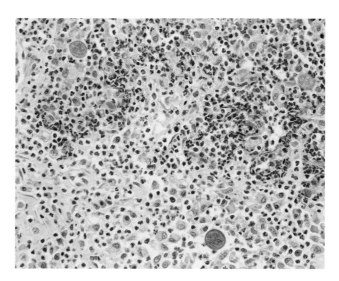

Figure 2.13   This is pyogranulomatous osteomyelitis due to coccidioidomycosis.

osteomyelitis (Figure 2.12). Extensive proliferation of new bone and granulation tissue is typical. In addition, there may be **sinuses** that allow pus to drain from the affected bone to the surface of the skin. Occasionally in bones with osteomyelitis, fragments of necrotic bone are present. If these fragments are small, they may be resorbed. However, if they are large, the usual response is to encapsulate them or force them to the body's surface through a sinus. These fragments of separated, necrotic bone are **sequestra**. Since sequestra are excellent harbors for bacteria, surgical removal usually speeds recovery.

   Pyogranulomatous and **granulomatous osteomyelitis** are additional forms of chronic osteomyelitis. They are usually caused by fungi and are often components of systemic mycosis. **Blastomycosis** and **coccidioidomycosis** are examples (Figure 2.13). Lesions are usually located in the epiphyses of long bones. Marked proliferation of new bone coupled with bony lysis, generally lead to firm swelling of the affected bone, which grossly can be confused with osteosarcoma.

Primary neoplasms of bone and cartilage occur in dogs, cats, and horses; malignant primary neoplasms are more frequent than benign ones in dogs and cats. Metastatic neoplasms in bone are infrequent in domestic animals, but in people, they are more frequent than primary bone tumors. A discussion of specific neoplasms is later in this chapter.

Obtaining a confirmed diagnosis of a skeletal neoplasm can be challenging. Clinical and pathologic examinations require **radiographic study** and **biopsy** to assure accurate diagnosis and prognosis. It can be difficult to obtain a diagnostic biopsy, so it is important to include superficial and deeper portions of the suspected neoplasm.

Joint Structure and Physiology

There are two major types of joints: **synarthroses**, which are fibrous connections between bones that move little and **diarthroses**, which are synovial joints that articulate. **Diarthrodial joints** are composed of bone ends, articular cartilage, and synovial lining and have a sleeve of connective tissue, ligaments, muscles, and tendons for support.

Adult articular cartilage is firm, pliable, and free of blood vessels and lymphatics. Besides chondrocytes, cartilage consists of collagen, glycosaminoglycans, proteoglycans, and water. Articular chondrocytes derive their nutrients from the synovial fluid. These chondrocytes maintain the matrix by the production of proteoglycans and structural collagen (types II and IX). In addition, chondrocytes produce metalloproteinases, which can degrade cartilage matrix. Therefore, to maintain the proper amount and character of the cartilage matrix, there is a balance between the production and destruction of the matrix components. The structural collagens provide a mesh-like framework, which maintains the shape and organization of the matrix. Type II collagen fibrils are the main component of the mesh and are spot-welded together by type IX collagen. The large complexes of glycosaminoglycans with proteoglycan side chains (called **aggrecan**), are packed around the collagen meshwork. These proteoglycans attract and bind water forming a hydrated gel. When opposing articular cartilage surfaces are compressed (i.e. during loading of a joint), a thin film of fluid is squeezed out of the cartilage matrix and accumulates on the opposing cartilage surfaces. This is called a "squeeze film" and along with synovial fluid, is an important lubrication mechanism for articular cartilage. Articular cartilage has a very limited capacity to repair itself once injury has occurred. Chondrocytes will proliferate when chronically injured, but their replication is ineffective at replacing a significant loss of cartilage. In addition, as an animal ages, the ability of chondrocytes to produce matrix declines; this also limits the reparative capacity of cartilage, especially in older animals, and contributes to the progression of degenerative joint disease.

The joint capsule is composed of an external fibrous layer and an inner synovial layer, usually referred to as the synovial membrane. The synovial membrane is composed of a ragged layer of synovial cells (synoviocytes) covering a layer of loose fibrovascular tissue; there is no basement membrane between the synoviocytes and the subjacent fibrovascular tissue. There are two types of synoviocytes based on structure and function: type A and type B synoviocytes. Type A synoviocytes are on the surface of the synovial membrane; they are phagocytic cells and possess many of the attributes of macrophages, such as the production of IL-1. Type B synoviocytes are spindle-shaped and usually at the interface with the adjacent fibrovascular tissue of the synovial membrane. Type B synoviocytes produce the hyaluronic acid found in the synovial fluid that is generated by the synovial membrane. This fluid is basically a transudate to which hyaluronic acid and other macromolecules have been added. It contains very few cells and does not contain fibrinogen. Synovial fluid functions to nourish the articular chondrocytes, maintain hydration of the cartilage matrix and provide boundary lubrication (primarily due to lubricin) to the joint surfaces. Therefore, for articular cartilage to maintain proper function, the synovial membrane and synovial fluid must be normal.

Basic Reactions of Joints to Injury

Tissue reaction to joint injury may involve the articular cartilage, the joint capsule, and/or the synovial membrane. **Chondromalacia** is the general term for softening and degeneration of articular cartilage. Microscopically, chondromalacia is characterized by eosinophilia of the matrix, dissolution and fissuring of the cartilage matrix, ulceration of the cartilage, chondrocyte necrosis, and proliferation of chondrocyte clusters (Figure 2.14). Additional changes that may occur with chronic joint injury include subchondral bone sclerosis, exudate accumulation on the articular surface, and growth of

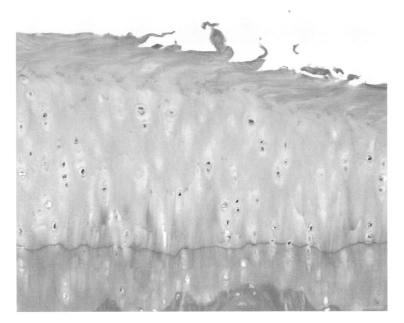

Figure 2.14   Chondromalacia with fissuring and eosinophilia of the cartilage matrix.

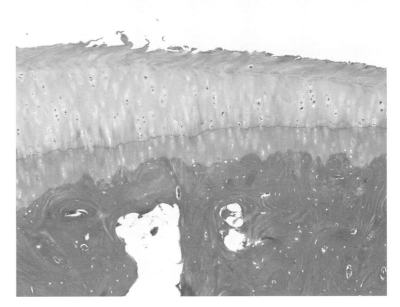

Figure 2.15   Chondromalacia with subchondral bone sclerosis. Note the formation of osteons resembling cortical bone.

fibrovascular tissue from the joint capsule over the articular surface. Injury to the joint capsule and synovial membrane stimulates changes that include inflammation, villous hyperplasia of synovial membrane, chondrification of synovial villi, fibrosis of the joint capsule, and formation of periarticular osteophytes. In addition, primary neoplasia of the joint capsule may develop, which typically is synovial cell sarcoma or histiocytic sarcoma (which are perhaps the same neoplasm).

Degenerative Changes in Articular Cartilage

Injured articular cartilage will typically lose components of the extracellular matrix as a result of degradation by matrix metalloproteinases, which results in eosinophilia of the matrix. In addition, as the matrix deteriorates, the cartilage will get thinner and begin to fissure. As the ability to generate a lubricating squeeze film is lost, the cartilage is worn away down to

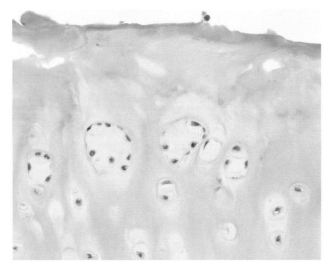

Figure 2.16   Proliferative clusters of chondrocytes (chondrones) along with eosinophilia and fissuring of the cartilage matrix.

subchondral bone. As this occurs, the subchondral bone receives a more direct, heavier load and responds with increased bone production, resulting in a dense subchondral plate that resembles cortical bone (Figure 2.15). An additional change that occurs is the proliferation of chondrocyte clusters, sometimes called **chondrones**; this apparently is an attempt at healing (Figure 2.16).

Inflammation of Articular Cartilage and Chondronecrosis

Since adult articular cartilage has no blood supply, exudate is not generated within the cartilage. However, inflammation of the joint may result in the accumulation of exudate on the articular surface. Neonatal animals have cartilage canals that contain vessels in the AE complex, and therefore exudate associated with subchondral osteomyelitis may accumulate in these canals and damage the articular cartilage. Chronic inflammation can result in the organization of exudate on the articular surface and/or ingrowth of fibrovascular tissue over the articular surface from the synovial membrane; this is termed **pannus** (Figure 2.17). Chondrocytes may die as a result of injury from bacterial toxins and/or chemical mediators of inflammation. **Chondronecrosis** is characterized by eosinophilia of chondrocytes within lacunae or empty lacunae (Figure 2.18, b).

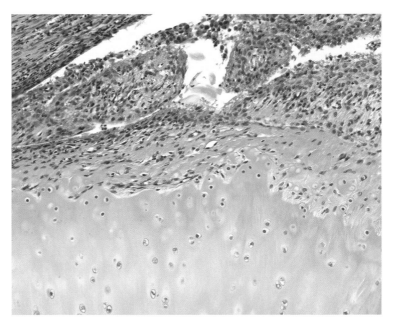

Figure 2.17   This is chronic arthritis with proliferation and ingrowth of fibrovascular tissue over the articular surface (pannus).

(a) (b)

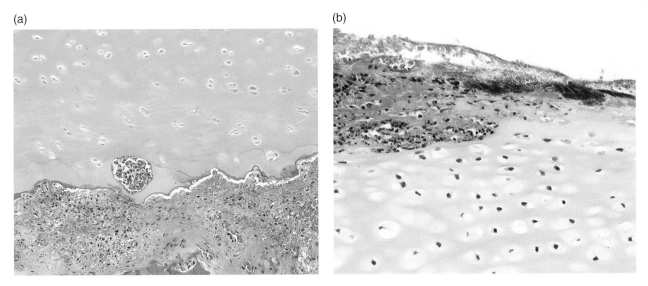

Figure 2.18 (a) Chondronecrosis and subchondral osteomyelitis. The cartilage lacunae contain eosinophilic remnants of necrotic chondrocytes. (b) This is arthritis with a bacterial biofilm along with necrosuppurative exudate, chondronecrosis and chondrolysis.

Inflammation of the Synovial Membrane and Joint Capsule

Synovitis, inflammation of the synovial membrane, is fairly common and can vary in severity and type of exudate; it can also be a component of more generalized arthritis or osteoarthritis. Fibrinous, purulent, pyogranulomatous, and lymphoplasmacytic exudates are the most common types encountered. It is interesting to note that many times cytologic preps of the synovial fluid from an inflamed joint will contain numerous pmns, but a biopsy of the associated synovial membrane will not; this presumably is because the pmns transmigrate out of the synovial vessels into the joint cavity rather rapidly. Chronically inflamed joints will commonly have **synovial villous hyperplasia**, characterized by finger-like projections of the synovial membrane covered with multiple layers of proliferative synoviocytes (Figure 2.19). Occasionally some of these villi will undergo metaplastic transition to cartilage (**chondrification**) or bone and may become loose objects within the joint (joint mice); when extensive, the condition is termed **synovial chondromatosis**. In addition, **fibrosis** of the joint capsule and proliferation of expansive fibrovascular tissue (pannus) may occur in certain forms of chronic synovitis and arthritis. Also, **periarticular osteophytes** may form at the attachment site of the joint capsule to the periosteum; when severe, these can fuse together to cause ankylosis of the joint.

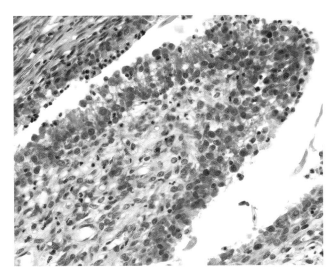

Figure 2.19 This is chronic synovitis with a substantial infiltrate of pmns and fibroblasts, along with synovial villous hyperplasia. Note the multiple layers of proliferative synoviocytes covering the villous structure.

Diseases of Bone

There are many diseases that primarily affect the skeleton, and many of these are diagnosed clinically via radiography and at necropsy. Only a subset of skeletal diseases is typically evaluated or primarily diagnosed via biopsy. This subset is the focus of the discussion that follows.

Developmental Disorders and Anomalies

The range of congenital and developmental skeletal disease is large, and causes are numerous, including genetics, toxins, nutrition, hormones, metabolic defects, and infectious agents. Some skeletal lesions are not apparent at birth but manifest as the animal develops.

Osteochondrosis

This is an important condition that develops in the sites of endochondral ossification in young, male, rapidly growing, large breeds of dogs, cattle, horses, pigs, chickens, and turkeys. Articular–epiphyseal complexes and growth plates are affected. The cartilage becomes focally thickened and is prone to fracture. This produces clefts in the cartilage; when these lesions occur in articular cartilage, a flap may break loose, and this is termed **osteochondrosis dissecans (OCD)** (Figure 2.20a, b). OC may cause transient or permanent lameness, which begins in the first year of life. Articular lesions are common in the shoulder and elbow joints and also occur on the lateral and medial condyles of the femur.

The pathogenesis of articular lesions may be different than that for the physeal lesions; in either location, OC is basically a defect in endochondral ossification. In affected animals, there is premature involution of vessels in the cartilage canals that supply nutrients to the growing cartilage of the AE complex. This results in focal ischemia and chondrocyte necrosis. Without viable chondrocytes to direct endochondral ossification, it is delayed at these necrotic foci, and the cartilage matrix fails to mineralize and be removed. However, endochondral ossification proceeds normally in cartilage adjacent to the necrotic foci, which results in focal accumulations of necrotic cartilage within the AE complex. If this accumulation of cartilage is large, it may break loose during use and form a flap of cartilage, which separates from the subchondral bone. The subchondral defect heals by granulation tissue and eventually fibrocartilage. Physeal lesions develop in association with delayed metaphyseal vessel penetration, but the cause of this is not known.

(a)

(b)

Figure 2.20   (a, b) Osteochondrosis dissecans starts out as a plug of necrotic cartilage due to premature closure of blood vessels. Eventually, the necrotic cartilage separates from the adjacent subchondral bone, resulting in an irregular articular surface.

(a) (b)

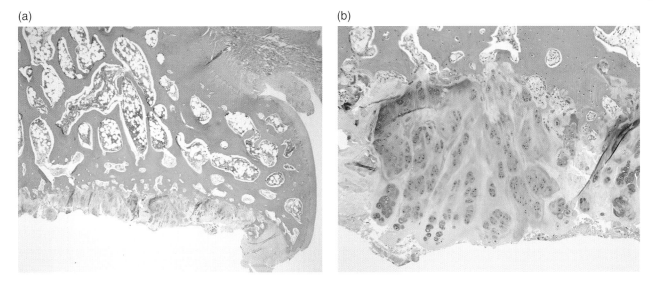

Figure 2.21 (a, b) Physeal dysplasia in a cat with fracture and separation of the femoral head (a). The physis is irregularly thickened and contains clusters of disorganized chondrocytes (b).

Other conditions thought to be part of the osteochondrosis syndrome in dogs are **ununited anconeal process**, **ununited medial coronoid process** of the ulna, **epiphysiolysis**, **retained cartilage core** of the distal ulna, and some cases of **slipped capital femoral epiphysis (epiphysiolysis)**.

Physeal Dysplasia in Cats

This is a syndrome recognized in young adult cats in which the physes are thickened and contain clusters of disorganized chondrocytes. The proximal femoral physes in affected cats are prone to fracture, resulting in separation of the femoral head. Overweight male cats are at increased risk of femoral head separation (Figure 2.21a, b).

Chondrodysplasia

Chondrodysplasia is usually an inherited condition that is manifest in young animals. There are many specific types of chondrodysplasia, but all are abnormalities of cartilage, which lead to abnormal endochondral ossification and secondary bone deformations.

Achondroplastic dwarfism is common in some breeds of dogs, i.e. bulldogs, bassets, Pekinese, etc. and cattle, i.e. Hereford and Angus. These animals are short-legged with short wide heads and protruding lower jaws (prognathism). The forehead protrudes and the maxillae are distorted. The head is often disproportionately large. The defect is likely in epiphyseal chondroblastic growth and maturation, causing inadequate endochondral bone growth.

Pseudoachondroplastic dysplasia occurs is miniature poodles and is evident in the first few weeks of life. The endochondral bones are short and have bulbous ends; cartilage of the epiphyses droop over the edges of the metaphyses. Chondrocytes vary in size and growth zones are irregular. Ossification is multifocal.

Chondrodysplasia occurs **in Alaskan malamutes**. This is short-limbed, disproportionate dwarfism that is an autosomal recessive inherited disease. Lesions are most severe in the distal radius and ulna. The affected growth plates have changes similar to those in rickets, but there is no evidence of Ca, P, or vitamin D deficiency. Excess matrix is formed in the proliferative zone of the growth plates, and this causes the growth plates to be thickened. Affected dogs also have hypochromic macrocytic anemia.

Chondrodysplasia in Norwegian Elkhounds is another form of short-limbed dwarfism, but the vertebral bodies are also short. The growth plates are narrowed due to a decrease in the thickness of the proliferative zone. Chondrocytes contain multiple vacuoles that are filled with glycosaminoglycans.

Osteochondromatosis (Multiple Cartilaginous Exostoses)

This is a developmental abnormality in which there are multiple chondro-osseous protuberances that extend out from the cortex of affected bones (Figure 2.22a, b). In dogs and horses, they occur in young animals, are usually close to the physes and continue to grow until the animal reaches skeletal maturity. These protuberances are shaped like a mushroom with a

(a) (b)

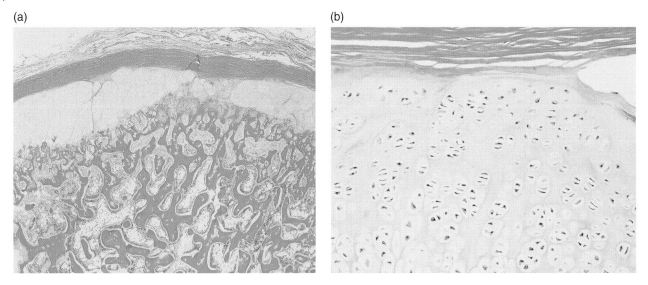

Figure 2.22   (a, b) Osteochondroma. This is composed of a stem of trabecular bone covered with a cap of hyaline cartilage and fibrous tissue.

cap of hyaline cartilage mimicking a normal growth plate upon a stem of bone. Feline osteochondromas are considered to be neoplasms (not developmental abnormalities) because they have a different presentation and course; they occur in adult cats, have a random distribution, progressively grow and may develop malignant characteristics.

Hyperostotic Diseases of Bone

This group of diseases has hyperostosis with little or no inflammation as a significant lesion. The hyperostosis that occurs has a similar microscopic appearance in all of these conditions. Some have known causes but others do not.

Hypertrophic (Pulmonary) Osteopathy

This is an enigmatic condition that occurs in several species, especially humans, dogs and horses. It is characterized by hyperostosis of the appendicular skeleton, especially the distal long bones, metatarsal and metacarpal bones, secondary to chronic disease, especially intrathoracic and intra-abdominal masses. Grossly, the affected limbs are thickened due to accumulation of edematous mesenchymal tissue in the deep fascial planes and a substantial layer of woven periosteal new bone (Figure 2.23a, b). Microscopically, the layer of periosteal new bone is similar to woven bone that forms in other conditions with trabeculae oriented perpendicular to the cortical surface.

The pathogenesis of HPO is unclear, but the bony lesion will resolve if the thoracic/abdominal mass is removed. Severing the vagus nerve will also cause remission.

Canine Hepatozoonosis

Infection with *Hepatozoon americanum* will stimulate cortical hyperostosis in dogs that closely resembles Hypertrophic Osteopathy. The distribution of the lesions tends to be on the proximal long bones and axial skeleton. The organisms are located in skeletal muscle, not in the bone.

Hyperostoses of Nutritional Origin

As mentioned earlier, hypervitaminosis A and D will cause hyperostosis.

Hyperostoses of Unknown Cause

Canine craniomandibular osteopathy (CMO or "Lion Jaw") is a disease of unknown etiology but likely has a genetic basis since most cases occur in Scottish and West Highland white terriers. It has a very characteristic gross appearance with hyperostosis primarily on the mandibles, temporal, and occipital bones. Microscopically, it is characterized by spicules of woven bone perpendicular to the cortical surface. The periosteal surface of the new bone is fairly cellular with

(a) (b)

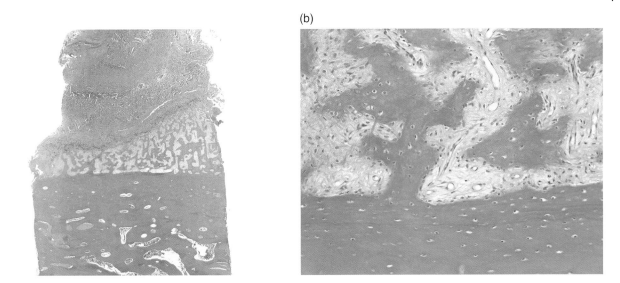

Figure 2.23   (a, b) Hypertrophic pulmonary osteopathy. This is composed of a layer of hyperostotic bone on the periosteal surface of an appendicular bone.

osteoblasts and a few pmns and lymphocytes. It is usually bilateral, but may be unilateral. It typically occurs in young dogs (4–7 months) causing pain when eating. Periods of progression and regression may be followed by complete remission at 11–13 months of age.

Canine Panosteitis is, despite the name, a typically non-inflammatory, self-limiting disease of long bones that occurs in young dogs (5–12 months of age), especially German Shepherds. Usually one limb is affected and there is no swelling or heat at the affected site although pain can be elicited by palpation. Lameness disappears and reappears in a different limb with eventual recovery. Diagnosis is usually made by radiography and therefore the lesion is rarely biopsied. Radiographically, the typical change is focal areas of increased radiodensity within the medullary cavity of the diaphysis. Microscopically these radiodense foci are composed of fibrovascular tissue that contains woven bone; there is no accumulation of exudate in these foci. In the resolving phase, the woven bone is remodeled into trabecular bone. The cause is not known.

Inflammatory Diseases of Bone

Inflammatory disease of bone is typically caused by an infectious agent, usually bacteria but occasionally fungi. As mentioned earlier, routes of infection are through the blood stream (hematogenous), a contaminated penetrating wound, or direct extension from an adjacent soft tissue infection. In addition, there are a few inflammatory bone diseases for which the cause is not known.

Osteomyelitis Caused by Bacterial Infection

Osteomyelitis in the A/E complex or metaphysis is the usual lesion caused by hematogenous bacterial infection in young animals, especially those with impaired immunity, such as failure of passive transfer. Although the diagnosis is usually made clinically by radiography, the lesions are fairly far advanced by the time radiographic changes are evident. Osteolysis with destruction of the adjacent cartilage, along with osteonecrosis and accumulation of fibrinopurulent exudate and fibrovascular tissue are typical at this stage. Agents involved vary somewhat with the species of animal affected. In foals, infection is commonly due to *Streptococcus* sp., *Rhodococcus equi*, *Salmonella* sp. and possibly *Actinobacillus equuli*. Osteomyelitis due to equine rhodococcosis usually will also have numerous macrophages containing bacteria and cell debris as a feature (Figure 2.24a, b). Neonatal osteomyelitis due to bacterial infection is relatively uncommon in puppies and kittens, but infection with *Streptococcus* sp., *Staphylococcus* sp., or coliforms should be considered.

(a)

(b)

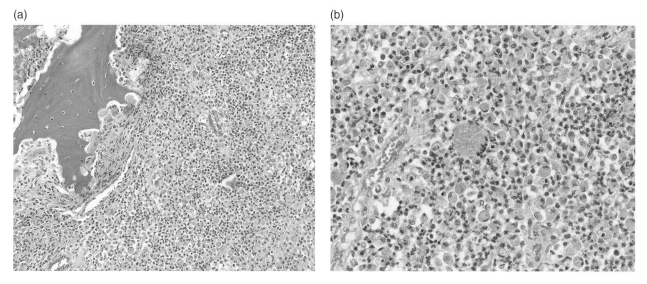

Figure 2.24   (a, b) Chronic pyogranulomatous osteomyelitis in a foal due to infection with *Rhodococcus equi*. Note the numerous macrophages, many of which contain bacteria.

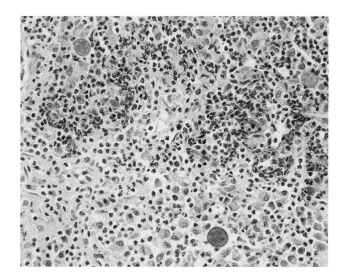

Figure 2.25   This is pyogranulomatous osteomyelitis due to coccidioidomycosis.

Osteomyelitis Caused by Fungal Infection

Fungal infection of bone is usually caused by one of the dimorphic fungi, *Blastomyces dermatitidis*, *Coccidioides immitis*, or *Histoplasma capsulatum*. There is a geographic distribution to these agents, but they typically cause a multisystemic infection in young adult animals. The osseous lesions produced are similar for all and are composed of pyogranulomatous exudate containing few to many organisms, osteolysis, and proliferation of new bone, which frequently results in a mass resembling a neoplasm (Figure 2.25).

Canine Metaphyseal Osteopathy (Canine Hypertrophic Osteodystrophy)

This is an idiopathic inflammatory disease of growing dogs, especially large and giant breeds. Swelling and hyperthermia of the metaphysis of long bones occur with pain, lameness, and pyrexia. As the disease progresses, the ends of affected bones are markedly thickened by an enlarged periosteum and by deposition of periosteal woven bone and cartilage (Figure 2.26a, b). The distal radius and ulna are usually affected. The microscopic appearance is characteristic and includes hemorrhage, necrosis of osteoblasts and an infiltrate of pmns at the chondro-osseous junction of the metaphysis along with

(a)

(b)

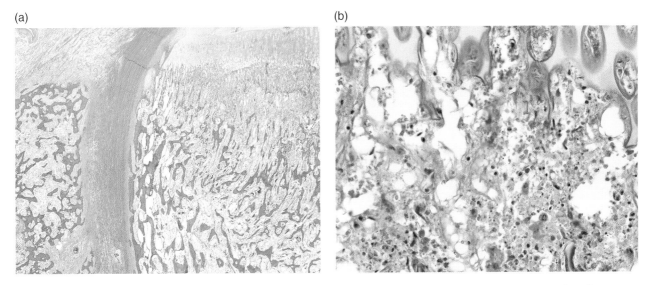

Figure 2.26   (a, b) Canine metaphyseal osteopathy. This is characterized by necrotizing inflammation of the metaphysis and hyperostosis on the adjacent cortical surface.

periosteal new woven bone. The lesions usually resolve and the bone resumes its normal contour. However, occasionally a case will be severe enough to result in angular deformity of the limb. It has long been suspected that some infectious agent is the cause but none has been consistently documented.

Osteonecrosis and Bone Infarction

Several diseases have osteonecrosis as a feature, including osteomyelitis due to bacterial infection and expansile neoplasms of bone that cause ischemia. However, the conditions described next are diseases in which osteonecrosis is the primary lesion.

Necrosis of the Femoral Head and Legg–Calve–Perthes Disease

Necrosis of the femoral head is fairly common in dogs. It can be due to **traumatic separation** of the femoral head, or it can be seen as an idiopathic condition termed **Legg–Calve–Perthes Disease (LCPD)**. Traumatic separation can occur in any animal, but LCPD only occurs in miniature-breed dogs. In LCPD, clinical signs develop at about four to eight months of age and are usually unilateral. The pathogenesis probably involves occlusion of venous drainage from the femoral head, perhaps as a result of a transient joint effusion. Experimental tamponade of the coxofemoral joint will produce femoral head necrosis. Dogs resistant to LCPD have intra-osseous veins, but susceptible dogs have many veins in the sub-synovium, which are susceptible to occlusion by increased intra-articular pressure. Whether due to traumatic separation or LCPD, the microscopic appearance of the femoral head is the same. This is characterized by osteonecrosis and necrosis of the marrow. If vascular supply is re-established, then osteoclast and osteoblast progenitor cells will move in and initiate resorption of the necrotic bone along with production of new bone upon the necrotic trabecula (Figure 2.27a–d). At this stage, it is common for the femoral head to cave in and cause irregularity in the overlying articular surface.

Bone Infarction

This is focal osteonecrosis due to ischemia secondary to a variety of causes such as thrombosis, thermal injury, or loss of the periosteum due to trauma. In dogs and cats, it is frequently associated with an expanding mass in the medullary cavity, such as lymphoma. In addition to the primary cause, the typical microscopic features are osteonecrosis, necrosis of the adjacent marrow, and depending on the duration; there may be osteolysis coupled with new bone production upon the necrotic bone (Figure 2.28a, b).

(a)

(b)

(c)

(d)

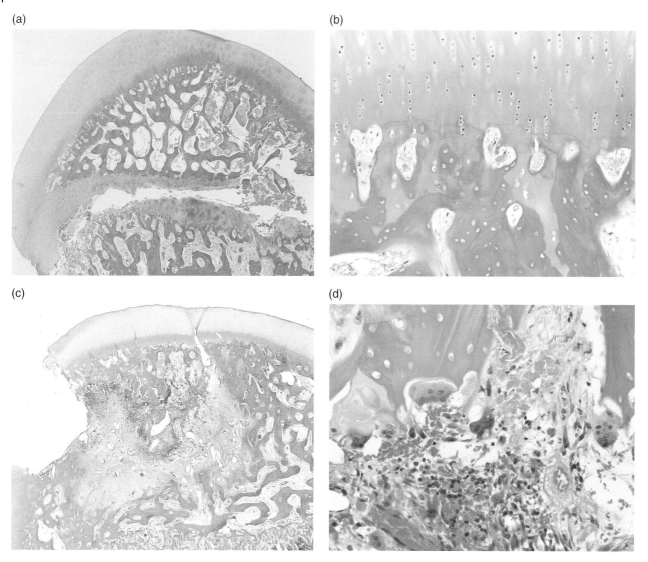

Figure 2.27   (a, b) Traumatic separation of the proximal femoral physis resulting in osteonecrosis of the femoral head. (c, d) Necrosis of the femoral head in a dog. Vascular perfusion has been restored, which has resulted in partial removal of necrotic bone and collapse of the head.

Neoplasia of Bone

Osteoma

This is a benign tumor of well-differentiated bone. Grossly, it is discrete and hard. Osteoma occurs most commonly in horses (especially on the rostral end of the mandible), but is rare in other species; they tend to be on the head and mandible (Figure 2.29). The characteristic microscopic appearance is a nodule of well-differentiated bone surrounded by fibrous tissue.

Osteosarcoma

Osteosarcoma (OS) is the most common type of primary bone tumor in dogs and cats. With respect to dogs, it usually occurs in mature males of large and giant breeds. OS most commonly occurs in the **metaphysis of long bones in very characteristic locations,** the proximal humerus, distal radius, distal femur, and distal tibia. It also occurs in the skull and occasionally in extraskeletal sites, such as the mammary gland and the intestine. OS usually arises in the medullary cavity of the metaphysis and expands and/or infiltrates through the cortex; when this occurs, a marked proliferative response ensues, which results in periosteal hyperostosis (**"Codman's triangle"**). Also, there are two types of OS that

(a)

(b)

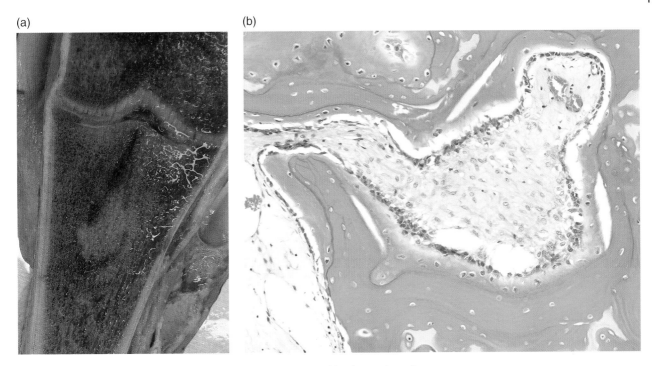

Figure 2.28   (a, b) Bone infarct. Necrotic bone has been covered with a layer of new bone.

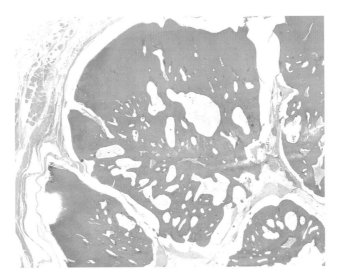

Figure 2.29   This is an osteoma on the maxillary gingiva of a dog. It is a circumscribed mass composed of well-differentiated bone.

start in the periosteum instead of the medullary cavity – periosteal OS and parosteal OS, which are discussed in more detail below. In addition to location, classification of OS as to subtype is based on the microscopic appearance and relative proportion of the extracellular matrix components, osteoid, cartilage, and fibrillar collagen. However, since different areas of the same OS can have substantially different proportions of these extracellular matrix components, it may be a bit artificial to classify OS based on the proportion of extracellular matrices. This variation is one thing to bear in mind when determining a subtype, especially with a small biopsy. An additional subtype of OS, the **telangiectatic OS**, contains blood-filled cavities and somewhat resembles hemangiosarcoma; however it is distinguished from hemangiosarcoma by the presence of osteoid produced by the neoplastic cells, and the blood-filled cavities are lined by neoplastic osteoblasts, similar to the rest of the neoplasm. Telangiectatic OS is considered to be the most aggressive of the osteosarcoma subtypes. **Metastasis occurs early**, usually to the lungs; therefore, the diagnosis of OS warrants a poor long-term prognosis.

There is some evidence that OS of the maxilla or mandible in dogs is somewhat slower to metastasize than OS of the appendicular skeleton.

Osteoblastic OS (Figure 2.30)
Chondroblastic OS (Figure 2.31)
Fibroblastic OS (Figure 2.32)
Telangiectatic OS (Figure 2.33a, b)
Giant cell OS (Figure 2.34)
Periosteal OS (Figure 2.35)
Parosteal OS (Figure 2.36)
Extraskeletal OS

Chondroma

Chondroma is a benign tumor of well-differentiated cartilage and is rare.

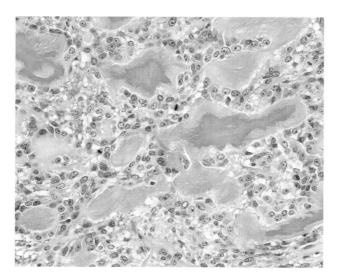

Figure 2.30 Osteoblastic osteosarcoma in a dog. Neoplastic pyriform to spindle osteoblasts produce globular to trabecular aggregates of osteoid.

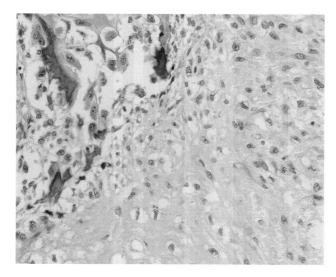

Figure 2.31 Chondroblastic osteosarcoma in a dog. Although the neoplastic osteoblasts are producing trabeculae of osteoid, there is also a significant production of cartilage.

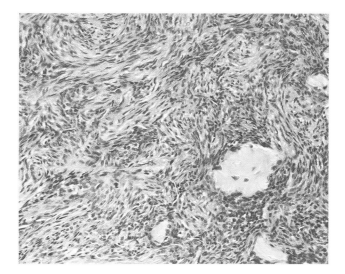

Figure 2.32   Fibroblastic osteosarcoma. Neoplastic cells have a spindle morphology, are aligned in intersecting bundles and produce collagenous extracellular matrix in addition to osteoid.

(a)   (b)

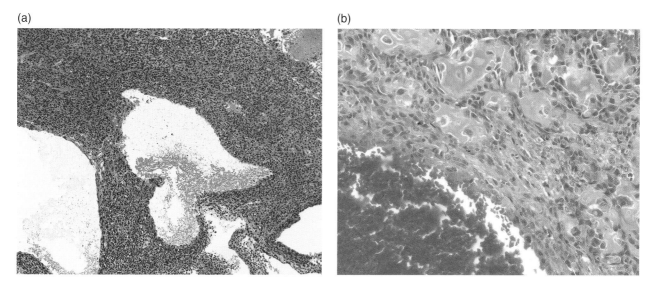

Figure 2.33   (a, b) Telangiectatic osteosarcoma. There are multiple blood-filled cavities lined by neoplastic osteoblasts, which produce aggregates of osteoid.

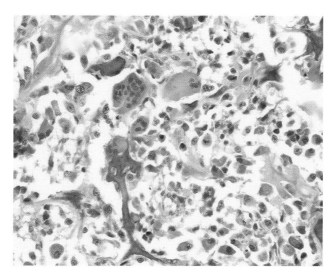

Figure 2.34   Giant cell osteosarcoma. These contain numerous multinucleate cells that somewhat resemble osteoclasts.

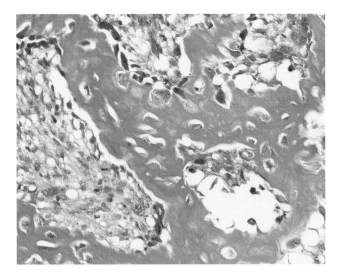

Figure 2.35   Periosteal osteosarcoma. This form of osteosarcoma has features similar to osteoblastic intramedullary osteosarcoma but develops on the periosteal surface of a bone.

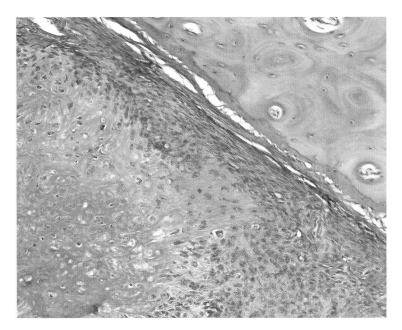

Figure 2.36   Parosteal osteosarcoma. This form of osteosarcoma develops in the soft tissue adjacent to the periosteum.

Chondrosarcoma

Chondrosarcoma (CS) occur with some frequency in dogs and sheep. They develop most commonly in the **head** (especially in the **nasal cavity**), **ribs**, and **axial skeleton**. CS is locally invasive but metastasizes later than osteosarcoma. Grossly, CS are large, multilobular masses composed of translucent cartilage. Microscopically, they may be very well differentiated, but they will often have anisocytosis and anisokaryosis with multiple cells within a single lacuna. The mitotic index is typically low to moderate; the presence of any mitotic figures is considered an indication of malignancy (Figure 2.37a–d).

Multilobular Tumor of Bone

Multilobular tumor of Bone is a distinctive neoplasm that most commonly occurs in the skull and mandible, primarily in dogs. They have been reported to occur in other bone locations, but this is uncommon. It is a slowly progressive, locally invasive neoplasm that may transform into osteosarcoma. It recurs following removal in about 50% of cases. Also, it may

(a)

(b)

(c)

(d)

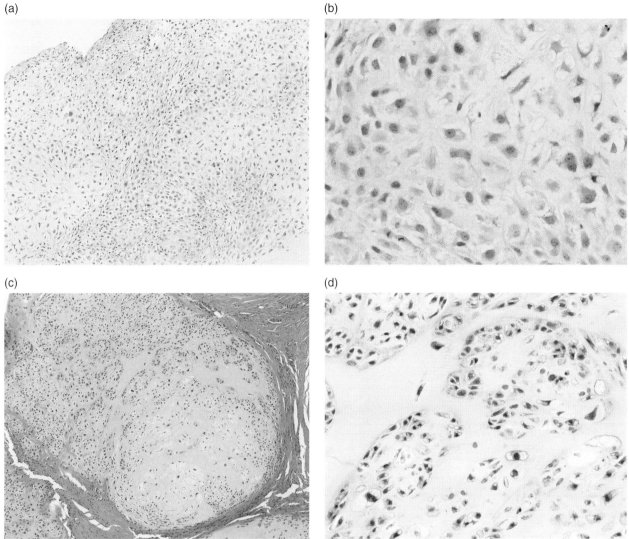

Figure 2.37 (a, b) Chondrosarcoma. Neoplastic chondrocytes are aligned in sheets and lobules, are round to stellate, and located within lacunae separated by a substantial amount of pale basophilic extracellular matrix. (c, d) Neoplastic chondrocytes are round to angular and are located within lacunae separated by a substantial amount of pale basophilic extracellular matrix.

metastasize, especially to the lungs. It is composed of lobules of cartilage and/or bone that are separated by fibrovascular septa. Centers of lobules often mineralize and undergo endochondral ossification (Figure 2.38a, b). These cause clinical disease referable to their location in the.

Osteochondroma
Osteochondromas This condition has already been discussed.

Giant Cell Tumor
Giant cell tumor is an uncommon, aggressive tumor of mesenchymal cells (Figure 2.39a, b).

Multiple Myeloma
Multiple myeloma (plasma cell tumors within the marrow cavity) occurs in the marrow cavity in dogs and typically causes a focal area of osteolysis.

(a)

(b)

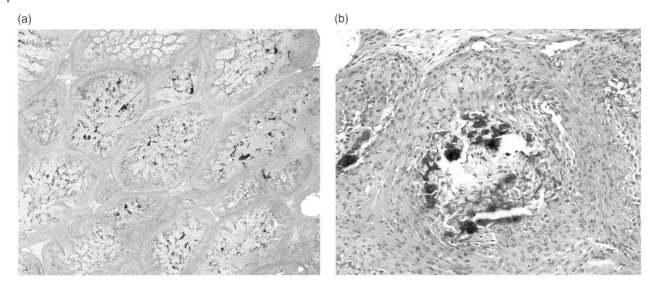

Figure 2.38 (a, b) Multilobular tumor of bone. This is composed of circumscribed lobules of cartilage, the centers of which undergo endochondral ossification.

(a)

(b)

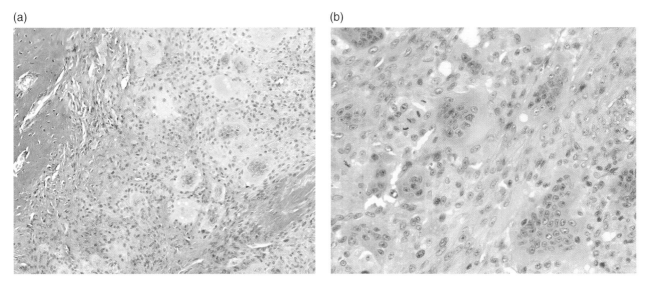

Figure 2.39 (a, b) Giant cell tumor of bone. These are composed of numerous multinucleate giant cells.

Chordoma

Chordoma is a mesenchymal neoplasm derived from a remnant of the notochord. They may occur anywhere in the spine, but we see them most commonly in the tail (Figure 2.40a, b). They are composed of large round to polyhedral cells with markedly vacuolated cytoplasm (physaliferous cells).

Hemangiosarcoma

Hemangiosarcoma will occasionally occur in bone, especially in the medullary cavity; when it does, the microscopic appearance is similar to hemangiosarcoma in other organs, such as the spleen. The main differential diagnosis is telangiectatic osteosarcoma.

Ossifying Fibroma

These are uncommon masses that occur most commonly in the rostral mandible of young horses. Basically, these consist of the proliferative, well-differentiated fibrous tissue expected in a fibroma, with the addition of trabecula of

(a)

(b)

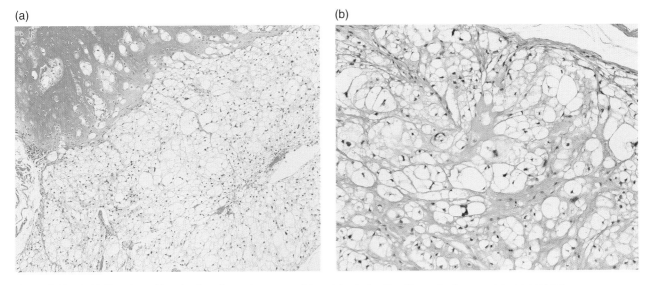

Figure 2.40   (a, b) Chordoma. Neoplastic cells are large round to polyhedral cells with markedly vacuolated cytoplasm (physaliferous cells).

(a)

(b)

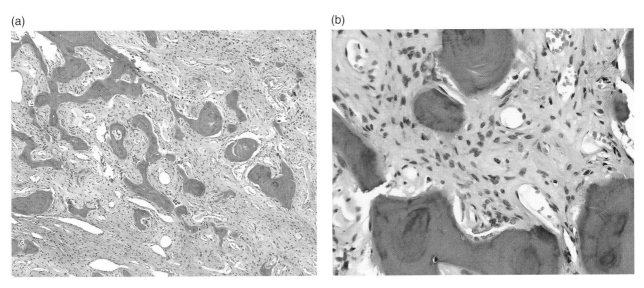

Figure 2.41   (a, b) Ossifying fibroma. These consist of well differentiated fibrous tissue as expected in a fibroma, with the addition of trabecula of well differentiated metaplastic bone.

well-differentiated metaplastic bone. The bone trabecula are typically oriented perpendicular to the surface of the mass, much like hyperostotic bone would be (Figure 2.41a, b).

Diseases of Joints

Osteochondrosis Dissecans

This condition is discussed in more detail in the Diseases of Bone section. However, OCD is the form of osteochondrosis that results in defects in articular cartilage. This is a result of necrosis and failure of endochondral ossification in the Articular/Epiphyseal complex, with subsequent fracture of a cartilage flap within the joint.

(a) (b)

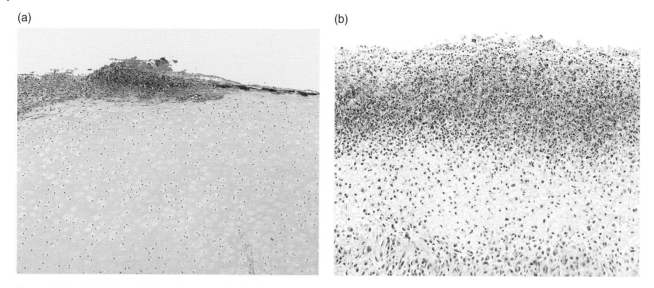

Figure 2.42   (a) This is arthritis with a bacterial biofilm along with necrosuppurative exudate, chondronecrosis, and chondrolysis. (b) This is the synovium in a joint with arthritis due to a bacterial infection. The ulcerated surface of the synovium is a layer of granulation tissue covered with a layer of fibrinopurulent and necrotic.

Infectious Arthritis due to Bacteria

This is typically caused by bacterial infection from either a penetrating wound into the joint or bacteremia. *Staphylococcus* sp., *Streptococcus* sp., and *E. coli* are common organisms that cause purulent to fibrinopurulent arthritis associated with a penetrating wound into the joint, which is the usual route of infection in adult animals. The same set of bacteria, along with some others (*R. equi, A. equuli* in foals), may infect one or more joints through the bloodstream, which is the more common route in young animals and is frequently associated with osteomyelitis (Figure 2.42a, b).

Lyme Disease

Infection with *Borrelia burgdorferi* can cause arthritis as a component of Lyme disease. This is a blood-borne infection transmitted by *Ixodes* sp. ticks. The microscopic lesion is lymphoplasmacytic synovitis.

Autoimmune and Immune-Mediated Arthritis

This is a set of uncommon, noninfectious forms of arthritis that are most prevalent in dogs and cats and frequently involve multiple joints (polyarthritis). Some group these as "erosive" or "non-erosive" based on the amount of articular cartilage involvement that is present. Members of the erosive group tend to have **pannus** as a feature, which is what causes cartilage erosion (Figure 2.43a–c). Probably most members of this group have fibrinous to fibrinopurulent inflammation in the early phase but then progress to lymphoplasmacytic inflammation in the chronic phase. Preferential involvement of certain joints is characteristic of different members of this group. Included here are rheumatoid arthritis, feline polyarthritis, polyarthritis of Greyhounds, and systemic lupus erythematosus.

Chronic Osteoarthritis

This is a very common condition in domestic animals, especially older animals. It may develop as a long-term result of conformational abnormalities, joint trauma, a variety of joint infections, and immune-mediated diseases, as essentially an end-stage condition. Regardless of the initial injury, the lesions that occur and characterize chronic osteoarthritis are very similar. These include joint capsule fibrosis, synovial villous hyperplasia, articular cartilage degeneration and loss, chondrone formation, subchondral bone sclerosis, pannus, and periarticular osteophyte formation. When infectious agents such as bacteria are the initial cause, there is frequently an infiltrate of lymphocytes, plasma cells, and possibly pmns within the synovium.

(a)

(b)

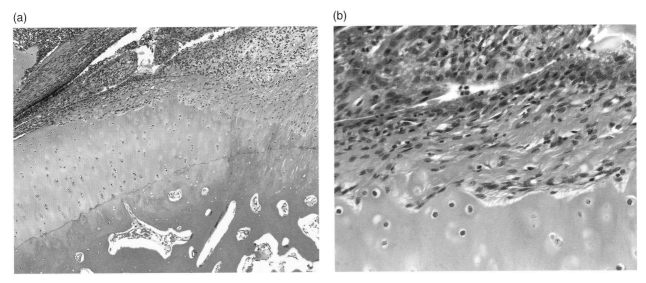

(c)

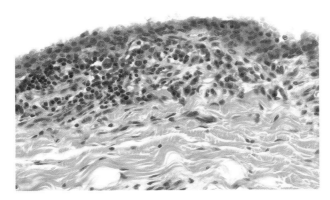

Figure 2.43   (a) This is chronic lymphoplasmacytic arthritis with articular cartilage destruction due to pannus formation. (b, c) Pannus formation destroying the articular cartilage. Also, there is a marked infiltrate of lymphocytes and plasma cells along with hyperplasia of the synoviocytes in the synovium.

Neoplasms of Joints

Histiocytic sarcoma of the joint capsule (Figure 2.44a–c) and **synovial sarcoma** (Figure 2.45a, b) are the two most common malignant neoplasms that arise in or around the joint in dogs. These may appear grossly and microscopically similar and be difficult to differentiate. Grossly, synovial sarcoma and histiocytic sarcoma of the joint capsule surround the joint, fill the joint cavity and may invade into bone, muscle, and tendon sheaths on both sides of the affected joint. Microscopically, the neoplastic cells are aligned in sheets, are round to spindle-shaped, have one or more round to oval nuclei, abundant eosinophilic cytoplasm, and discernible cell borders. The neoplastic cells of histiocytic sarcoma are presumed to originate from interstitial dendritic cells within the joint capsule and are typically positive for CD18 and Iba 1 via immunohistochemistry.

Synovial myxoma is reported to be the most common benign neoplasm of joints; these form nodules in the synovial membrane composed of loose stellate cells separated by pale extracellular matrix. They are most common in the stifle and interphalangeal joints, and although they do not metastasize, they are invasive into adjacent bone and along fascial planes (Figure 2.46a, b).

The usual set of sarcomas that occur in animals (fibrosarcoma, rhabdomyosarcoma, liposarcoma, peripheral nerve sheath tumors, etc.) can also occur in and around the joint capsule.

(a)

(b)

(c)

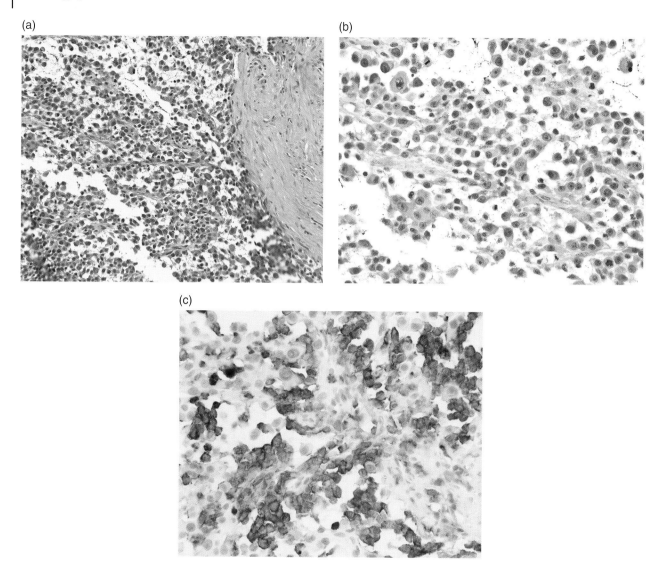

Figure 2.44 (a–c) Histiocytic sarcoma of the joint capsule. The neoplastic cells are variably sized, round to spindle cells. They are positive for CD18.

(a)

(b)

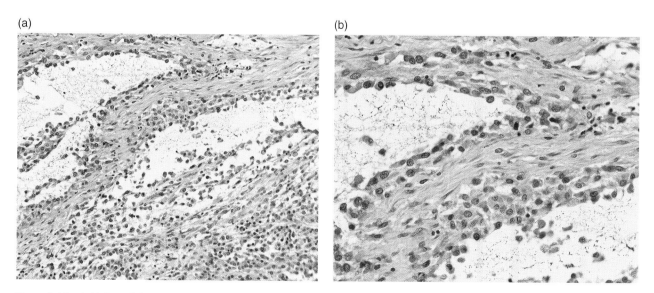

Figure 2.45 (a, b) Synovial sarcoma.

(a) (b)

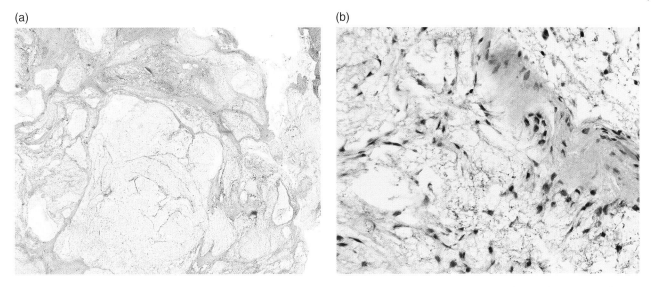

Figure 2.46   (a, b) Synovial myxoma. These form nodules in the synovial membrane composed of loose stellate cells separated by a pale extracellular matrix.

References and Additional Readings

Bingel, S.A., Sande, R.D., and Wight, T.N. (1985 Oct). Chondrodysplasia in the Alaskan malamute. Characterization of proteoglycans dissociatively extracted from dwarf growth plates. *Lab Invest.* 53 (4): 479–485. PMID: 4046558.

Chomel, B. (2015). Lyme disease. *Rev. Sci Tech.* 34 (2): 569–576. https://doi.org/10.20506/rst.34.2.2380.

Craig, L.E. (2001). Physeal dysplasia with slipped capital femoral epiphysis in 13 cats. *Vet. Pathol.* 38 (1): 92–97. https://doi.org/10.1354/vp.38-1-92.

Craig, L.E., Julian, M.E., and Ferracone, J.D. (2002). The diagnosis and prognosis of synovial tumors in dogs: 35 cases. *Vet. Pathol.* 39 (1): 66–73. https://doi.org/10.1354/vp.39-1-66.

Craig, L.E., Krimer, P.M., and Cooley, A.J. (2010). Canine synovial myxoma: 39 cases. *Vet. Pathol.* 47 (5): 931–936. https://doi.org/10.1177/0300985810369903.

Dernell, W.S., Straw, R.C., Cooper, M.F. et al. (1998). Multilobular osteochondrosarcoma in 39 dogs: 1979–1993. *J. Am. Anim. Hosp. Assoc.* 34 (1): 11–18. https://doi.org/10.5326/15473317-34-1-11.

Greenwell, C.M., Brain, P.H., and Dunn, A.L. (2014). Metaphyseal osteopathy in three Australian Kelpie siblings. *Aust. Vet. J.* 92 (4): 115–118. https://doi.org/10.1111/avj.12162.

Maxie, M.G. (2016). Chapter 2 – Bones and joints. In: *Jubb, Kennedy and Palmer's Pathology of Domestic Animals*, 6e, vol. 1 (ed. L. Craig, K. Dittmer and K. Thompson), 16–163.

Panciera, R.J. and Ewing, S.A. (2003). American canine hepatozoonosis. *Anim. Health Res. Rev.* 4 (1): 27–34. https://doi.org/10.1079/ahrr200348.

Roush, J.K., Manley, P.A., and Dueland, R.T. (1989). Rheumatoid arthritis subsequent to *Borrelia burgdorferi* infection in two dogs. *J. Am. Vet. Med. Assoc.* 195 (7): 951–953. PMID: 2793577.

Schumacher, H.R., Newton, C., and Halliwell, R.E. (1980). Synovial pathologic changes in spontaneous canine rheumatoid-like arthritis. *Arthritis Rheum.* 23 (4): 412–423. https://doi.org/10.1002/art.1780230404.

Thornburg, L.P. (1979). Infantile cortical hyperostosis (Caffey–Silverman syndrome). Animal model: craniomandibular osteopathy in the canine. *Am. J. Pathol.* 95 (2): 575–578. PMID: 377993; PMCID: PMC2042330.

Craig, L. and Thomson, K. (2020). Chapters 9 – Tumors of joints. In: *Tumors in Domestic Animals*, 5e (ed. D. Meuten), 337–355. and Chapter 10 – Tumors of bones (ed. L. Craig, K. Dittmer, and K. Thompson), 356–424.

3

Pathology of the Skin

Joseph S. Haynes

Department of Veterinary Pathology, Iowa State University, Ames, IA, USA

Introduction

Skin is the largest organ of the body, and biopsies of skin lesions make up a substantial portion of surgical pathology specimens. Also, the diversity of lesions is substantial, ranging from developmental abnormalities to inflammatory and autoimmune diseases to neoplasia. This chapter does not contain all of the skin diseases that occur in veterinary medicine but attempts to present the most common skin lesions and diseases that are submitted to a veterinary surgical pathology service.

Specimen Preparation and Fixation

The best skin specimens for general evaluation are those taken with a 3–4 mm round biopsy punch and fixed in 10% neutral buffered formalin. This type of specimen is more desirable than a linear incisional specimen, because it does not twist during fixation and is more easily oriented for sectioning. At trim in, this type of specimen should be cut in half with the plane of section parallel to the length of the hair follicles. For cutaneous masses that are large enough, a section should be taken through the center of the mass, extending from one surgical margin to the opposite margin; then at least one additional section should be taken at a right angle to the initial section from the remaining fragments of the specimen. At minimum, this approach will provide several points along the deep margin and four reasonably spaced points on the lateral margins for evaluation of surgical clearance.

Basic Reactions of Skin to Injury

Skin diseases are characterized by a combination of gross and microscopic lesions, which are basic reactions to injury; many of these are listed in the table below (Table 3.1). Any particular lesion is not necessarily diagnostic for a particular disease. However, a group of lesions and the pattern in which they occur, especially microscopically, will frequently lead to diagnosis. Therefore, recognizing these lesions and patterns is essential to making a correct diagnosis.

Inflammation of the Skin: Dermatitis

Dermatitis is common in all species but is nonspecific. It may be localized or generalized and can be caused by a multitude of agents including autoimmune processes. It may be primary or secondary and is frequently self-induced from scratching due to **pruritus**. Inflammation of the skin usually involves the dermis and epidermis.

Table 3.1 Terms used in describing microscopic skin lesions.

Vesicle – small (<0.5 or 1 cm), circumscribed elevation of epidermis caused by a pocket filled with clear serum in or immediately beneath the epidermis. They are also termed blisters. Similar larger lesions are blebs or bullae (>1 cm).

Pustule – superficial abscess. A vesicle that contains neutrophils, as well as serum.

Scales – bran-like flakes of imperfectly cornified superficial epidermis.

Crusts – partially adherent plaques made of dried accumulations of serum, blood, pus, epithelial and bacterial debris.

Erosions – partial loss of the epidermis.

Ulcer – loss of epidermis to and through the basement membrane.

Lichenification – an irregular thickening of the skin characterized by acanthosis, hyperkeratosis and hyperpigmentation in response to chronic irritation.

Scar – fibrous tissue replacing normal tissue injured by disease or injury. In skin these are often alopecic and depigmented.

Acanthosis – hyperplasia of epidermis, especially in the stratum spinosum with down growth and enlargement of rete ridges/pegs.

Pseudoepitheliomatous hyperplasia – pronounced acanthosis resembling a carcinoma. This is often found at margins of chronic focal inflammation and ulcers.

Orthokeratotic hyperkeratosis (Orthokeratosis) – excessive thickness or hyperplasia of the stratum corneum resulting in laminated normal appearing keratin layers that lack nuclei.

Parakeratotic hyperkeratosis (Parakeratosis) – excessive thickness or hyperplasia of the stratum corneum due to imperfect cornification of the stratum corneum with retention of nuclei.

Acantholysis – loss of cohesion between epidermal cells due to degeneration of desmosomes.

Spongiosis – intercellular edema in the epidermis; this may lead to vesicle formation.

Ballooning degeneration – intracellular edema or hydropic degeneration of epidermal cells.

Pigmentary incontinence – presence of melanin within the superficial dermis due to basal cell injury associated with interface dermatitis.

Microscopic Patterns of Cutaneous Inflammation

In microscopic diagnosis of skin diseases, it is important to recognize the precise location of the inflammatory reaction or pattern. Inflammatory skin disease can be classified into various patterns, depending on the location of the exudate and associated changes. Some of the important ones are superficial perivascular dermatitis, interface dermatitis, lichenoid dermatitis, nodular and/or diffuse dermatitis, folliculitis/furunculosis, vasculitis, intraepidermal vesicular/pustular dermatitis, subepidermal vesicular/pustular dermatitis and panniculitis. This is a useful classification scheme because certain diseases tend to cause a specific pattern of inflammation.

Superficial perivascular dermatitis has inflammatory cells primarily localized around blood vessels in the superficial dermis (Figure 3.1). It is the typical pattern in allergic skin disease. **Interface dermatitis** has inflammatory cells localized at the dermal-epidermal junction; it is the typical pattern in several autoimmune diseases such as discoid lupus erythematosus (Figure 3.2). **Lichenoid dermatitis** is characterized by a continuous layer of inflammatory cells in the superficial dermis adjacent to the epidermis (Figure 3.3). **Vasculitis** of the skin has exudate within the wall of the cutaneous vessels; this occurs with immune complex deposition as in systemic lupus erythematosus (Figure 3.4a, b). **Intraepidermal vesicular/pustular dermatitis** is characterized by the presence of vesicles or pustules within the epidermis; an example would be pemphigus foliaceus (Figure 3.5). **Subepidermal vesicular/pustular dermatitis** has vesicles or pustules below the epidermis. **Folliculitis** is inflammation of the hair follicles; if the follicle ruptures and the inflammation extends into the adjacent dermis, it is **furunculosis** (Figure 3.6a, b). **Panniculitis** is inflammation of the subcutaneous adipose tissue, which is usually granulomatous or pyogranulomatous.

Acute Dermatitis

The process of acute inflammation in the skin is similar to acute inflammation in other tissues. It begins with erythema and edema of the dermis. Blood and lymphatic vessels of the dermal papillae are dilated, and dermal collagen bundles are separated by serous exudation (also termed edema).

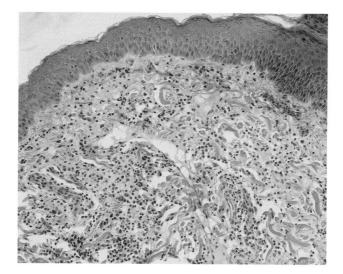

Figure 3.1 Superficial perivascular dermatitis. This pattern of inflammation is typical of allergic skin disease.

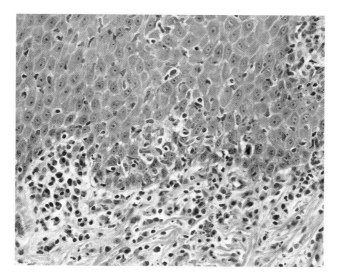

Figure 3.2 Interface dermatitis. This pattern of inflammation is typical of autoimmune skin diseases, such as discoid lupus erythematosus, in which the stratum basale is targeted.

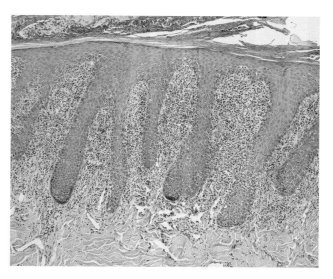

Figure 3.3 Lichenoid dermatitis. This pattern of inflammation is characterized by a continuous layer of inflammatory cells in the superficial dermis adjacent to the epidermis.

(a) (b)

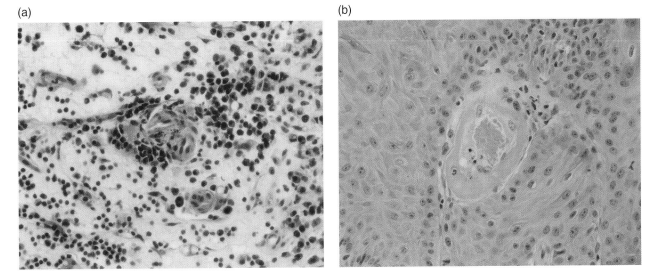

Figure 3.4   (a, b) Dermal vasculitis. This is leukocytoclastic vasculitis; the arteriolar wall is somewhat hyalinized with a smudged appearance and contains karyorrhectic cell debris.

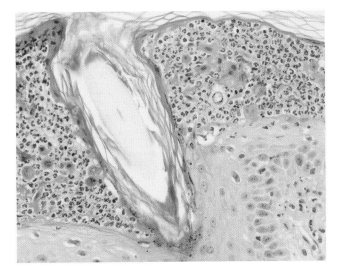

Figure 3.5   Intraepidermal Pustular dermatitis. This is pemphigus foliaceus with a subcorneal pocket of pus containing acantholytic keratinocytes.

(a) (b)

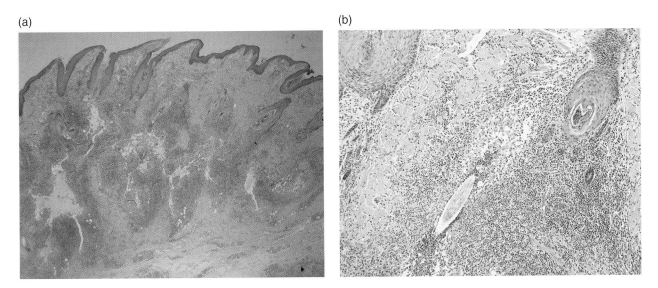

Figure 3.6   (a, b) Folliculitis and furunculosis. Folliculitis is characterized by exudate within the lumen or wall of the hair follicles. Furunculosis is characterized by exudate around and in place of ruptured hair follicles and fragments of hair.

If vesicles form, they may fill with leukocytes and become pustules, particularly if there is a bacterial invasion. Vesicles are often pruritic and rupture due to tension or self-inflicted trauma to relieve itching. Ruptured vesicles can expose deeper layers (erosions and ulcers) and ooze serum. Exudate from ruptured vesicles coagulates on the surface and forms crusts. Alopecia can occur due to self-trauma from scratching. The outcome of acute dermatitis depends on many factors. It may heal by re-epithelialization if ulceration is involved, it may lead to fibrosis and scarring, or, as often happens, it may lead to chronic dermatitis.

Chronic Dermatitis

Chronic dermatitis has a prolonged course and is characterized by dermal fibrosis, epidermal hyperplasia with acanthosis and hyperkeratosis, and infiltration by chronic inflammatory cells (lymphocytes, plasma cells, macrophages, mast cells, and possibly pmns). In fact, because of these epidermal changes, sometimes this is called **hyperplastic dermatitis** and may progress to lichenification (Figure 3.7). Atrophy of hair follicles and adnexal glands can also be seen in prolonged cases

Because chronic dermatitis tends to be stereotyped, the appearance of many chronic skin diseases is similar. Therefore, in order to diagnose the cause of clinical cases of dermatitis, acute and subacute lesions are more useful for arriving at an etiologic diagnosis if the lesion is biopsied.

Chronic dermatitis characterized predominantly by macrophages is properly termed **granulomatous dermatitis** or **pyogranulomatous dermatitis** (if neutrophils are also abundant) (Figure 3.8a, b). This type of reaction frequently involves the panniculus, dermis, and epidermis. Distinct granulomas or diffuse infiltration may occur. Grossly the skin may be nodular or ulcerated. Typical causes include foreign bodies such as grass awns, systemic mycotic agents, higher bacteria, and fragments of hair shafts.

Panniculitis is inflammation of the panniculus (subcutis) and is typically granulomatous or pyogranulomatous. It may be focal or diffuse. In chronic disease, subcutaneous tissue is replaced by fibrous connective tissue or diffuse granulomatous inflammation with sheets of macrophages or focal granulomas (Figure 3.9a, b). Panniculitis sometimes occurs because of nutritional reasons such as yellow fat disease of cats that is likely due to Vitamin E deficiency. In many cases, panniculitis is idiopathic.

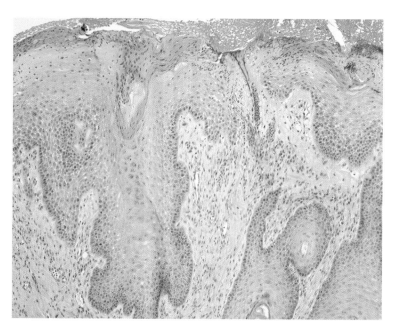

Figure 3.7 Hyperplastic dermatitis. There is marked hyperplasia of the epidermis (acanthosis) along with hyperkeratosis, dermal fibrosis, and a variable dermal infiltrate of inflammatory cells.

(a) (b)

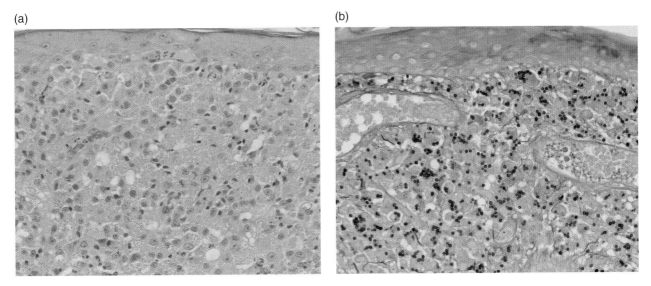

Figure 3.8   (a, b) Granulomatous dermatitis due to cutaneous histoplasmosis. GMS stain on right demonstrates these organisms.

(a) (b)

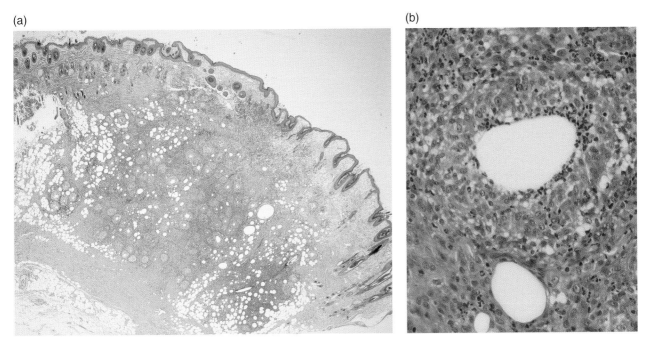

Figure 3.9   (a, b) Panniculitis. This is inflammation of the panniculus, which typically has granulomatous or pyogranulomatous exudate.

Abnormal Keratinization

Accumulation of excessive keratin (hyperkeratosis) is a very common reaction to cutaneous injury and can occur in a variety of diseases including chronic dermatitis, endocrine disease, nutritional abnormalities, and developmental abnormalities. It is considered to be a disruption of normal epidermal turnover and epidermopoiesis. Orthokeratotic hyperkeratosis (orthokeratosis) is the retention of superficial cornified epidermal cells that lack nuclei. Parakeratotic hyperkeratosis (parakeratosis) is the retention of abnormally cornified epidermal cells that retain their pyknotic nuclei (Figure 3.10a, b).

(a) (b)

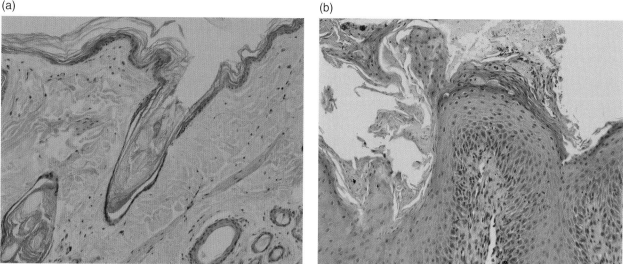

Figure 3.10 (a, b) Hyperkeratosis. There is orthokeratotic hyperkeratosis in the left image (a) and parakeratotic hyperkeratosis in the image on the right (b).

Alopecia

Lack of hair commonly occurs with skin injury or abnormal metabolism. The pattern and location of hair loss is indicative of certain diseases. The actual loss of the hair is either due to an abnormality in hair/hair follicle development, breakage of the hair shaft or epilation from trauma, atrophy of the hair follicle, or destruction of the hair follicle.

Abnormal Pigmentation

Increased or decreased accumulation of melanin are common lesions in several skin diseases. Hyperpigmentation occurs secondary to chronic injury to the skin, either focally or generalized. Loss of pigmentation is typically due to destruction of melanocytes and/or the cells of the stratum basale that contain melanin and is usually focal or multifocal. There are also developmental abnormalities of melanin production that may cause albinism or color-dilution mutant hair coat patterns.

Diseases of the Skin

Developmental Disorders and Anomalies of the Skin

Ichthyosis
This is a rare inherited disease reported in dogs and cats that is caused by defective keratin synthesis. It results in thick plate-like aggregates of keratin on the epidermal surface. There are typically fissures within the keratin plates, which result in a "fish scale" appearance. Microscopically, there is typically marked orthokeratosis, which may extend into hair follicle infundibula and acanthosis with ballooning degeneration (Figure 3.11a, b).

Primary Seborrhea
This occurs as an early-onset disease in several dog breeds. The secondary seborrheic disease may be due to parasitism, hormone imbalances, hypersensitivities, nutritional causes, environmental factors, etc. Whatever the cause, seborrhea is characterized by scaling and crusting often with a greasy texture. Because the epidermis is altered, the normal flora is altered, and normal microbial inhabitants are replaced by pathogens. Secondary bacterial infections are very common in seborrhea patients and frequently seborrheic dogs are infected with *Malassezia pachydermatis*, a yeast. Characteristic microscopic changes included scaling with parakeratosis, acanthosis, and often spongiosis. A common feature is the accumulation of parakeratotic caps or plugs within and on the rim of the follicular infundibulum.

(a)

(b)

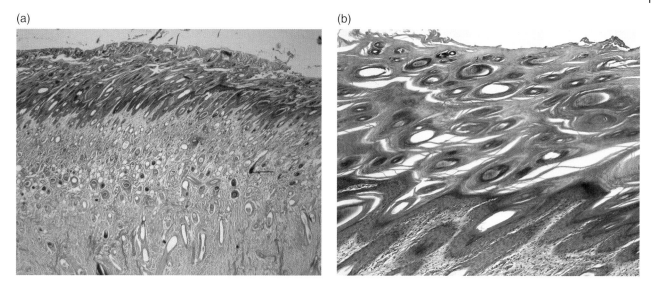

Figure 3.11 (a, b) Ichthyosis. There is marked orthokeratotic hyperkeratosis with formation of scale-like plates of keratin.

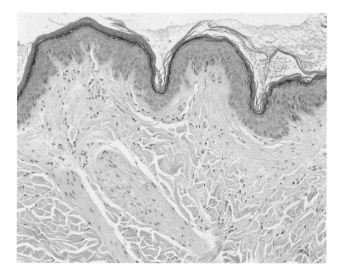

Figure 3.12 Hyperplastic dermatosis of West Highland White Terriers. Microscopically, there is marked acanthosis with scalloping of the deep epidermal margin.

Hyperplastic Dermatosis of the West Highland White Terriers

This is considered to be an extreme hyperplastic epidermal response to cutaneous injury unique to Wes Highland White Terriers. Injury from bacteria, such as *Staphylococcus* sp. and fungi, especially *M. pachydermatis*, have been implicated in initiating this condition. Microscopically, there is marked acanthosis with scalloping of the deep epidermal margin. In addition, there may be hyperplasia of sebaceous glands, and a variable dermal infiltrate of pmns, lymphocytes, and plasma cells (Figure 3.12).

Zinc Responsive Dermatosis

This disease occurs in Siberian Huskies and Alaskan Malamutes and may be due to an inherited defect in zinc absorption or metabolism. Characteristic changes include alopecia and scaling around the mucocutaneous junctions, nasal planum, and eyes. Microscopically, there is marked acanthosis with parakeratosis that extends into the hair follicle infundibula. Also, there is frequently a variable degree of inflammation with a dermal infiltrate of lymphocytes, plasma cells, and macrophages (Figure 3.13a, b).

(a)

(b)

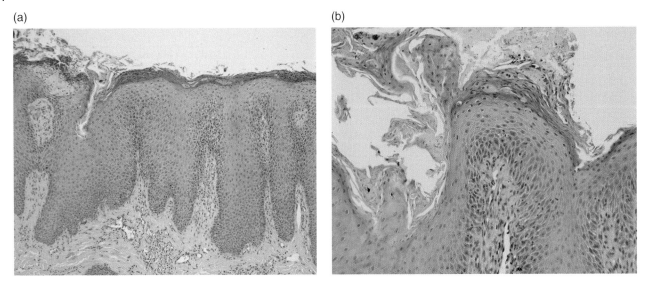

Figure 3.13   (a, b) Zinc-responsive dermatosis. There is marked acanthosis with parakeratotic hyperkeratosis.

Black-Hair Follicular Dysplasia and Color Mutant Alopecia

This is a condition in which the nonpigmented hair is normal, but the pigmented hair is very sparse. **Color mutant alopecia** occurs in several breeds, Dobermans, fawn Irish setters, and others, as a condition in which puppies are normal, but over the first year of life progressive alopecia develops often along with dermatitis. The microscopic changes are similar for both conditions; these consist of large clumps of melanin within the hair bulb, hair shaft, and keratin within the follicle. The follicles may be somewhat misshapen and lack hairs or may be in telogen or anagen phase (Figure 3.14).

Collagen Dysplasia

This is the term for the general category of disease that includes Ehlers–Danlos syndrome (man), dermatosparaxis (cattle), and cutaneous asthenia. Collagen dysplasias are characterized by different degrees of fragility of the skin and peripheral blood vessels and hyperextensibility of skin and joints in some cases depending on the enzymatic defects in collagen synthesis. Dogs, cats, mink, and man have autosomal dominant forms. Laxity and fragility of the skin lead to lacerations when

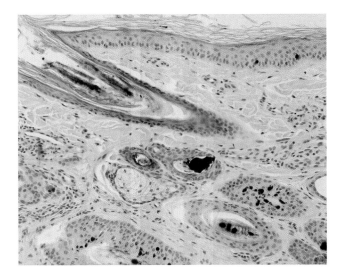

Figure 3.14   Color mutant alopecia. There are large clumps of melanin within the hair bulb, hair shaft, and keratin within the follicle. There is also modest hyperkeratosis with alopecia.

minimal force is applied. Frequent lacerations and poor wound healing are the typical presenting clinical complaint. Microscopically, the skin may appear to be normal, although occasionally, collagen bundles may be fragmented and lack orientation.

Degenerative, Atrophic, and Necrotizing Diseases of the Skin

Endocrine-Related Disease

Atrophic Dermatosis   Atrophic dermatosis can be local due to many processes or generalized due to senility or a variety of endocrine disturbances especially hypothyroidism, hyperadrenocorticism, and hyperestrogenism. Atrophic dermatosis is the typical diagnosis for skin changes, which include bilaterally symmetrical alopecia, epidermal thinning, dryness, fine wrinkles, and poor elasticity.

Endocrine dermatosis is characterized by loose and flaky hyperkeratosis, thin epidermis, follicular hyperkeratosis, atrophy of hair follicles and adnexa. Hair follicles are often empty or contain predominantly telogen hairs. The skin is also often hyperpigmented. Inflammation may be superimposed on the fundamentally altered skin making the diagnosis more difficult to make (Figure 3.15).

Hypothyroidism   Characteristic microscopic changes include atrophy of hair follicles and adnexa, normal to thick epidermis, hyperpigmentation, myxedema, and orthokeratotic hyperkeratosis. Hair follicles are usually in telogen phase or lack hair shafts and are filled with keratin.

Hyperadrenocorticism   Characteristic microscopic changes include orthokeratotic hyperkeratosis, a thin epidermis, atrophied hair follicles that are dilated and contain plugs of keratin (comedomes). Hair follicles are usually in telogen phase or lack hair shafts and occasionally contain aggregates of mineralized keratin. A distinctive feature is **calcinosis cutis**, in which mineral aggregates accumulate in the dermal collagen and the external root sheath of hair follicles (Figure 3.16a–c). Also, occasionally, there may be osseous metaplasia in areas of calcinosis cutis.

Hyperestrogenism   The microscopic changes are similar to hypothyroidism, with symmetrical alopecia, hyperkeratosis, variable-thickness epidermis, follicular hyperkeratosis, and hair follicles that are often empty or contain predominantly telogen hairs.

Growth Hormone Responsive Dermatosis   The microscopic changes are similar to those with the other endocrine abnormalities.

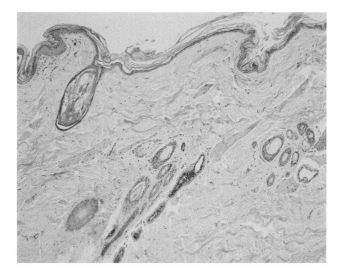

Figure 3.15   Atrophic dermatosis. There is moderate orthokeratotic hyperkeratosis, epidermal thinning, follicular hyperkeratosis, alopecia, and adnexal atrophy.

(a)

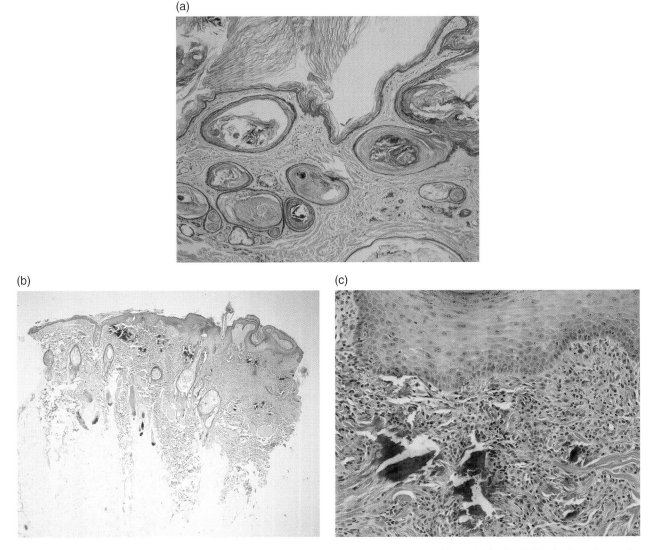

(b)

(c)

Figure 3.16 (a) Hyperadrenocorticism. There is moderate orthokeratotic hyperkeratosis, epidermal thinning, follicular hyperkeratosis, alopecia, and adnexal atrophy. (b) Hyperadrenocorticism with calcinosis cutis. In addition to follicular hyperkeratosis and alopecia, there are aggregates of mineral within the dermal collagen and occasionally within hair follicles. (c) There are aggregates of mineral within the dermal collagen, many of which are surrounded by granulomatous exudate.

Cyclical Flank Alopecia   This condition occurs in a variety of dog breeds and is characterized by bilaterally symmetrical alopecia of the flanks. Microscopically, there is orthokeratosis and follicular hyperkeratosis. The follicular hyperkeratosis has a somewhat distinctive pattern caused by the accumulation of laminated keratin that fills not only the follicular infundibulum but also fills dilated secondary follicular lumens, giving the appearance of a "foot" (so-called "Witch's foot") (Figure 3.17).

Superficial Necrolytic Dermatitis

This is a characteristic cutaneous lesion that occasionally develops in some dogs with chronic liver disease or glucagon-secreting pancreatic tumors. The pathogenesis of the skin lesion is not understood but is thought to involve hypoamino-acidemia. The classic "red, white, and blue" microscopic lesion is composed of a superficial layer of parakeratosis ("red"), a layer of epidermal edema in the stratum spinosum ("white"), and hyperplasia of the stratum basale ("blue") (Figure 3.18). Lesions are most common in areas of trauma, such as around the muzzle and on the footpads. This condition is the cutaneous component of the **hepatocutaneous syndrome.**

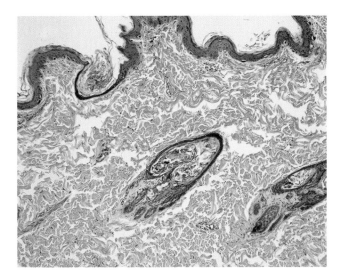

Figure 3.17   Cyclic flank alopecia. There is orthokeratotic and follicular hyperkeratosis. The follicular hyperkeratosis has a somewhat distinctive pattern caused by accumulation of laminated keratin that fills not only the follicular infundibulum but also fills dilated secondary follicular lumens, giving the appearance of a "foot" (so-called "Witches foot").

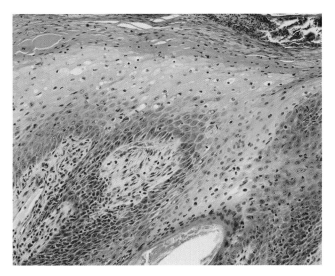

Figure 3.18   Superficial necrolytic dermatitis. The classic "red, white, and blue" microscopic lesion is composed of a superficial layer of parakeratosis ("red"), a layer of epidermal edema in the stratum spinosum ("white"), and hyperplasia of the stratum basale ("blue").

Toxic Epidermal Necrolysis

This is a severe cutaneous disease that is characterized by diffuse necrosis/apoptosis of the epidermis associated with modest dermal inflammation. This results in ulceration followed by substantial inflammation of the dermis (Figure 3.19). The pathogenesis is not clear, but it is thought to be due to cutaneous drug reaction that liberates toxic cytokines, especially TNF-α.

Cutaneous Infarction

This results in focal full-thickness necrosis of the skin, including the dermis. It may be secondary to vasculitis, thrombosis, or thermal or freezing injury (Figure 3.20).

Inflammatory Diseases of the Skin

Allergic Skin Diseases

Allergic skin disease is very common in cats and dogs. The various hypersensitivities are often incriminated, and while it is nice to cleanly split these out into the various types, many hypersensitivities are likely a combination of type I and type IV

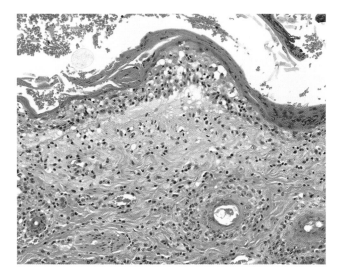

Figure 3.19   Toxic epidermal necrolysis. There is diffuse epidermal necrosis and apoptosis of keratinocytes.

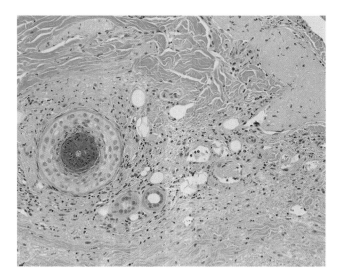

Figure 3.20   Cutaneous infarct due to thrombosis.

hypersensitivity. The typical microscopic lesion is superficial perivascular dermatitis. Secondary lesions from the self-trauma of scratching due to pruritus often complicate the diagnosis.

Classical **type I hypersensitivity (immediate type)** disease is mediated by mast cells (or basophils) and IgE. Lesions can be generalized without specific distribution. Transient dermal edema (wheals, hives, urticaria) with marked pruritus may be seen. Antigens that are incriminated in causing this type are pollens, endotoxin, ectoparasites, drugs (especially penicillin), food, insect bites, etc.

Delayed or type IV hypersensitivity (allergic contact dermatitis) must be distinguished from primary contact dermatitis. There is little if any dependence on antibody; cell-mediated immunity and not histamine release is the initial important event. Although the hypersensitivity is "delayed," dermatitis is often acute beginning as erythema and progressing to papules that itch and induce self-trauma that can lead to secondary pyoderma and eventually chronic dermatitis. T-lymphocytes and macrophages are the predominant inflammatory cells present.

Atopy   This is a genetically associated predisposition to type I hypersensitivity. Approximately 10% of small animal skin cases may be due to atopy. Affected animals contact the offending antigens through inhalation, ingestion, or percutaneously. Inhalation appears to be the most important route. The reaction occurs in the skin causing superficial perivascular dermatitis with edema, mast cells and eosinophils, pruritus, itching, scratching, and self-trauma (Figure 3.21a, b).

(a) (b)

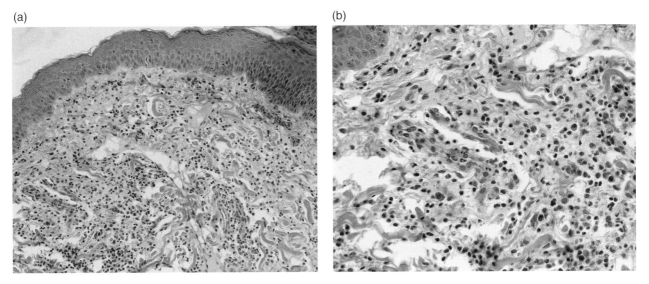

Figure 3.21 (a, b) Superficial perivascular dermatitis due to allergic skin disease. The perivascular infiltrate is composed of mast cells, eosinophils, lymphocytes, and plasma cells.

Canine Flea-Bite Hypersensitivity This form of allergic dermatitis is caused by a combination of Type I and Type IV hypersensitivity to flea salivary antigens. The microscopic appearance is similar to other forms of allergic dermatitis; depending on the duration, there is superficial perivascular to diffuse dermatitis with a variable infiltrate of eosinophils, mast cells, macrophages, lymphocytes, pmns, and plasma cells. In chronic cases, there is acanthosis and hyperkeratosis.

Allergic Contact Hypersensitivity This form of cutaneous hypersensitivity is caused by cutaneous contact with an allergen to which the animal has been previously sensitized. A variety of compounds have been associated with allergic contact hypersensitivity, including plants, environmental chemicals, and topically-applied drugs. Type IV hypersensitivity, characterized by a dermal infiltrate of lymphocytes and macrophages along with lymphocytic exocytosis and spongiosis of the epidermis is considered to be the basic reaction. However, the microscopic appearance can be somewhat variable and may also contain features of type I hypersensitivity, including a superficial dermal infiltrate of eosinophils and mast cells.

Feline Miliary Dermatitis

This form of allergic dermatitis is characterized by multifocal erosions or ulcers with serocellular crusts and superficial perivascular dermatitis. The inflammation is characterized by dermal edema, spongiosis and an infiltrate of eosinophils, mast cells, and lymphocytes (Figure 3.22a, b).

Feline Eosinophilic Plaque These are cutaneous nodular to plaque-like lesions that commonly occur on the ventral abdomen and medial thighs of cats and are considered to be a manifestation of allergic skin disease. Microscopically, there is typically acanthosis with epidermal mucinosis and spongiosis, along with a substantial dermal infiltrate of eosinophils, macrophages, lymphocytes, and plasma cells (Figure 3.23).

Feline Eosinophilic Granuloma (Feline Linear Granuloma, Feline Collagenolytic Granuloma) This is a fairly common lesion in cats, which may have one of several distribution patterns, including a raised linear or plaque-like lesion on the thighs. The characteristic microscopic features include a multifocal to diffuse dermal infiltrate of eosinophils, along with aggregates of hypereosinophilic collagen (flame figures) surrounded by a layer of degranulated eosinophils. Frequently, these aggregates of collagen are also surrounded by epithelioid macrophages and multinucleate giant cells, forming discreet granulomas (Figure 3.24a–c).

Canine Eosinophilic Granuloma Cutaneous eosinophilic granulomas are much less common in dogs than in cats, but when they occur, they have a microscopic appearance very similar to those in cats, with a dermal infiltrate of eosinophils, along

(a)

(b)

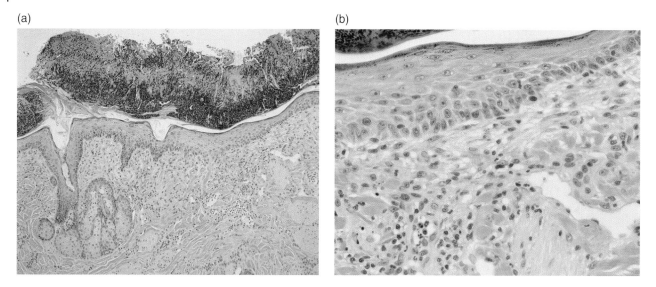

Figure 3.22 (a, b) Feline miliary dermatitis. There is multifocal to diffuse erosion with serocellular crusts, along with dermal edema and a perivascular dermal infiltrate of eosinophils, mast cells, and lymphocytes.

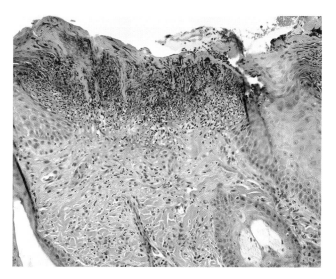

Figure 3.23 Feline eosinophilic plaque. There is typically acanthosis with erosion, ulceration, and spongiosis, along with a substantial dermal infiltrate of eosinophils, macrophages, lymphocytes, and plasma cells.

with aggregates of hypereosinophilic collagen (flame figures) surrounded by a layer of degranulated eosinophils, epithelioid macrophages and multinucleate giant cells (Figure 3.25a, b).

Equine Collagenolytic Granuloma This is the equine version of an eosinophilic granuloma and is microscopically very similar to eosinophilic granulomas in cats and dogs (Figure 3.26a, b).

Rabies Vaccine-Associated Vasculitis/Panniculitis This is a fairly common focal alopecic hyperpigmented lesion that occurs in dogs at the site of subcutaneous rabies vaccination. It is characterized by leukocytoclastic to cell-poor vasculitis in the panniculus and deep dermis that results in atrophy of adjacent hair follicles and adnexa along with hyalinization of dermal fibrous tissue. In addition, there are occasionally aggregates of lymphocytes along with scattered macrophages in the deep dermis and panniculus (Figure 3.27a–d).

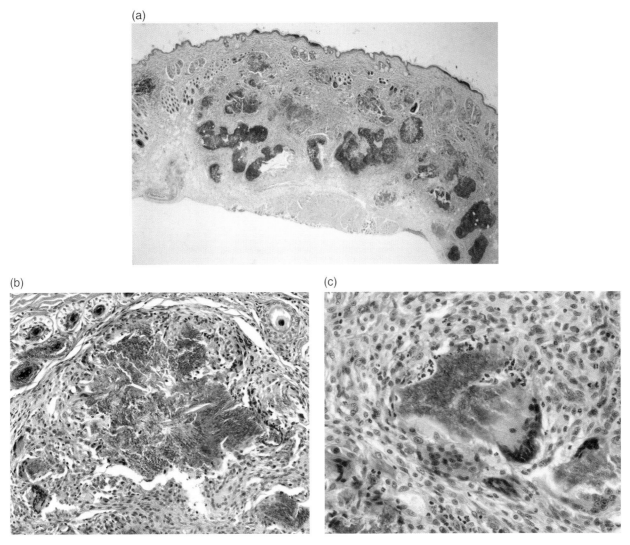

Figure 3.24   (a–c) Feline linear granuloma. There are multiple aggregates of fragmented and hyalinized collagen surrounded by epithelioid macrophages, multinucleate giant cells and scattered eosinophils.

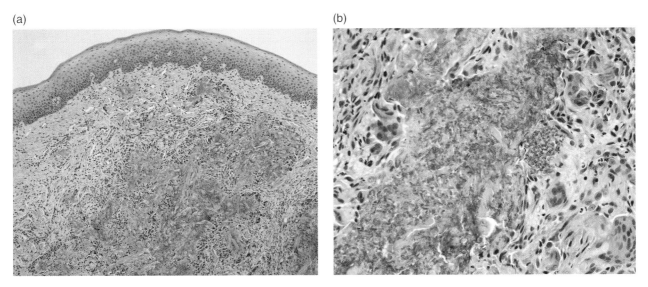

Figure 3.25   (a, b) Canine eosinophilic granuloma. Hyalinized and fragmented aggregates of collagen surrounded by epithelioid macrophages, multinucleate giant cells, and scattered eosinophils.

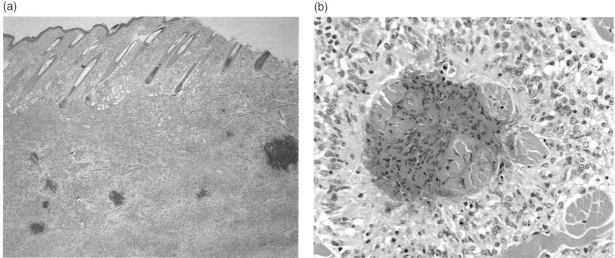

Figure 3.26 (a, b) Equine collagenolytic granuloma. Hyalinized and fragmented aggregates of collagen surrounded by epithelioid macrophages, multinucleate giant cells, and scattered eosinophils.

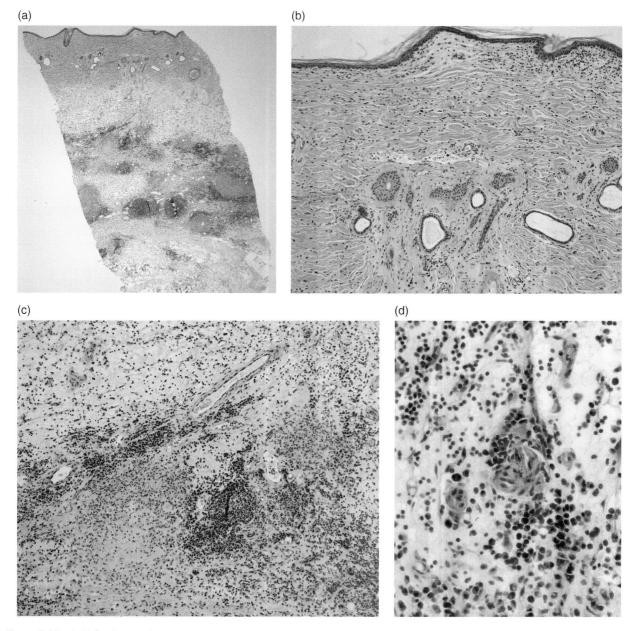

Figure 3.27 (a, b) Rabies vaccine-associated vasculitis/panniculitis. This is characterized by aggregates of lymphocytes, plasma cells, and macrophages along with leukocytoclastic to cell-poor vasculitis in the panniculus and deep dermis, which results in atrophy of adjacent hair follicles and adnexa along with hyalinization of dermal fibrous tissue. (c, d) There is a marked perivascular lymphocytic/plasmacytic infiltrate along with leukocytoclastic or cell-poor vasculitis.

Autoimmune Skin Diseases

Immune-mediated diseases of the skin include the relatively common hypersensitivities discussed earlier and autoimmune diseases. In the latter group, animals produce an immune response, usually antibody, to specific parts of their own skin causing a variety of lesions including blisters, bullae, pustules, ulceration, and dermatitis. The cause of the immune response directed against self-antigens is not known.

Pemphigus is a term that refers to one of several similar diseases in which antibody is directed against components of the epidermis such as the glycocalyx between cells, desmosomes, and/or basement membranes. Antibody binding stimulates plasminogen activator secretion that causes the epidermal cells to separate from one another (acantholysis), resulting in the formation of vesicles, blisters, bullae, or pustules. Erosions and ulcers result. The location of the reaction in the skin varies on the subtype of pemphigus. Grossly, vesicles, bullae, erosions, and ulcers may be seen along with hyperemia. Lesions in pemphigus vulgaris, for example, may appear first on mucous membranes of the oral cavity, but other types of pemphigus may have no involvement of the mucous membranes.

Pemphigus Vulgaris   Microscopically, in pemphigus vulgaris there is a separation of keratinocytes at the junction between the stratum basale and the stratum spinosum forming suprabasilar clefts. Vesicle formation between basal and prickle cell layers results; this leaves a single layer of basal epithelium attached to the basement membrane. These vesicles rupture readily to form erosions and ulcers with trauma or infection. There is also often lymphocytic interface dermatitis.

Pemphigus Foliaceus   This disease is characterized by intra- or subcorneal pustules containing pmns, occasionally eosinophils, and individual and/or rafts of acantholytic keratinocytes. Acantholysis may be present along the base of the pustule. Frequently, there are crusts on the surface that contain degenerate pmns and scattered acantholytic keratinocytes (Figure 3.28). Foci of acantholysis with pustule formation may also be present in the hair follicle epithelium. There is usually a moderate perivascular to diffuse infiltrate of lymphocytes, pmns, macrophages, and plasma cells within the superficial dermis. **Facially predominant pemphigus foliaceus** is a form of PF that has the additional feature of a lichenoid band of inflammatory cells in the superficial dermis (Figure 3.29a, b).

Pemphigus Erythematosus   This form of pemphigus, which is limited to the face, has features of both pemphigus foliaceus and discoid lupus erythematosus. Characteristic microscopic features include intra- or subcorneal pustules containing pmns, occasionally eosinophils, and individual and/or rafts of acantholytic keratinocytes along with lymphocytic interface dermatitis with foci of spongiosis, basal cell apoptosis, and pigmentary incontinence.

Bullous Pemphigoid   This is a very rare condition that is characterized by formation of subepidermal bullae as a result of autoimmune attack on the attachment site of basal keratinocyte to the basement membrane.

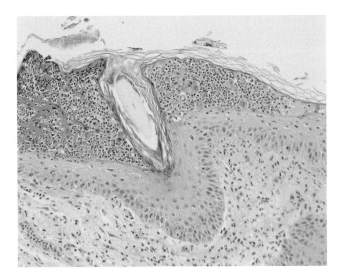

Figure 3.28   Pemphigus foliaceus. Subcorneal pustule containing acantholytic keratinocytes.

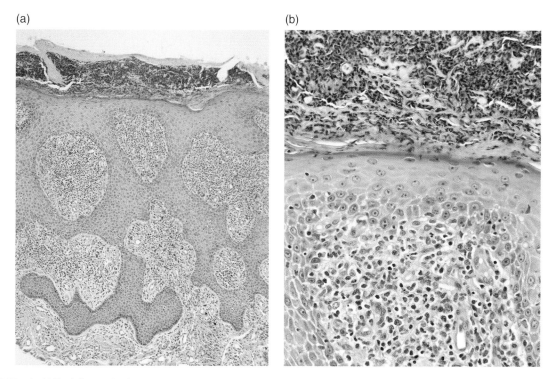

Figure 3.29 (a, b) Facially predominant pemphigus foliaceus. In addition to subcorneal pustules with acantholytic keratinocytes, there is a lichenoid band of lymphocytes, plasma cells, and macrophages in the superficial dermis.

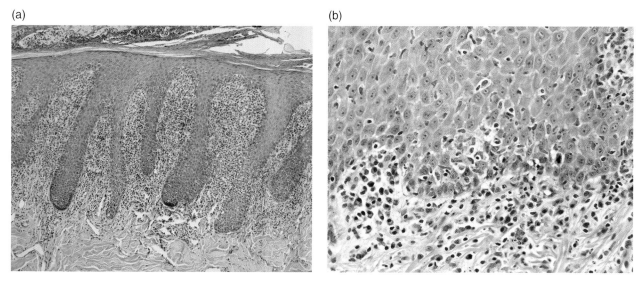

Figure 3.30 (a, b) Discoid lupus erythematosus. This is lymphoplasmacytic interface dermatitis with spongiosis, scattered apoptotic keratinocytes in the stratum basale, and pigmentary incontinence.

Discoid Lupus Erythematosus This is a fairly common autoimmune skin disease in which lymphocytes attack the stratum basale. Lesions are most common on face and muzzle and typically consist of symmetrical areas of scaling, crusts, and depigmentation. Characteristic microscopic features include interface lymphoplasmacytic dermatitis along with spongiosis and scattered apoptotic keratinocytes in the stratum basale and pigmentary incontinence (Figure 3.30a, b).

Exfoliative Cutaneous Lupus Erythematosus of the German Shorthair Pointer This is a disease that occurs in young German Shorthair Pointers, which is characterized by parakeratosis, lymphocytic interface dermatitis with spongiosis and scattered apoptotic keratinocytes in the stratum basale (Figure 3.31).

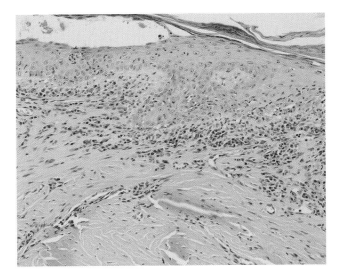

Figure 3.31 Exfoliative cutaneous lupus erythematosus of German Shorthair Pointers. There is parakeratosis with scattered apoptotic cells and spongiosis in the stratum basale, along with a lymphoplasmacytic interface infiltrate.

Erythema Multiforme This is a cutaneous lesion that is considered to be a T-cell mediated hypersensitivity targeting epidermal cells. It may be initiated by any one of multiple events, such as drug administration, neoplasia, and certain infections. The typical microscopic change is multifocal keratinocyte apoptosis with lymphocyte satellitosis throughout all layers of the epidermis. In addition, there is typically an interface infiltrate of lymphocytes and macrophages, along with spongiosis of the stratum basale and occasionally pigmentary incontinence. Lesions may be severe enough to result in ulceration (Figure 3.32).

Lupoid Onychitis This disease is characterized by lymphocytic interface inflammation of the nail bed that results in crumbling and loss of one or more claws. Microscopically, there is lymphocytic interface inflammation, spongiosis, and scattered apoptotic keratinocytes in the stratum basale (Figure 3.33).

Psoriasiform–Lichenoid Dermatosis This unusual condition occurs primarily in Springer Spaniels and is characterized by proliferative hyperkeratotic cutaneous plaques. Microscopically, there is marked acanthosis with intraepidermal pustules and a substantial lichenoid dermal infiltrate of lymphocytes, plasma cells, and macrophages (Figure 3.34).

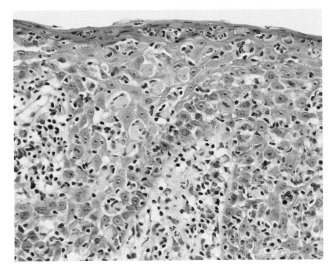

Figure 3.32 Erythema multiforme. There is multifocal keratinocyte apoptosis with lymphocyte satellitosis throughout all layers of the epidermis, along with an interface infiltrate of lymphocytes and macrophages and spongiosis of the stratum basale with modest pigmentary incontinence.

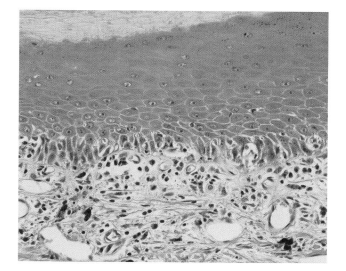

Figure 3.33 Lupoid onychitis. There is lymphocytic interface inflammation, spongiosis, and scattered apoptotic keratinocytes in the stratum basale of the nail bed.

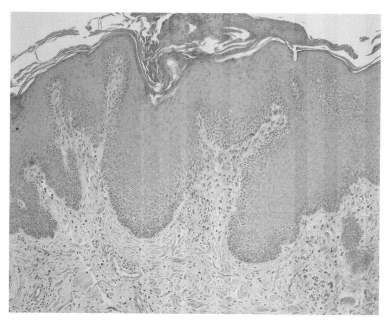

Figure 3.34 Psoriasiform-Lichenoid dermatosis. There is marked acanthosis with intraepidermal pustules and a substantial lichenoid dermal infiltrate of lymphocytes, plasma cells, and macrophages.

Uveodermatologic Syndrome This condition occurs in multiple breeds of dogs, but especially in the Artic breeds such as Akitas, Samoyeds, Malamutes, and Huskies. This is generally considered to be an autoimmune disease in which melanin-containing cells are the target. The skin lesions are characterized by marked depigmentation, especially of the muzzle, associated with a substantial lichenoid infiltrate of macrophages, many of which contain melanin (melanophages). The ocular lesion is primarily granulomatous uveitis/endophthalmitis with numerous melanophages (Figure 3.35a, b).

Idiopathic Equine Pastern Leukocytoclastic Dermatitis This is a chronic dermatitis with leukocytoclastic vasculitis, which typically occurs on the nonpigmented skin of the pasterns in adult horses. It is thought that UV radiation has a role in this condition, and there may be an immune-mediated component as well. Microscopically, there is marked acanthosis and parakeratotic hyperkeratosis with serum lakes. Many small vessels in the superficial dermis have thickened, somewhat

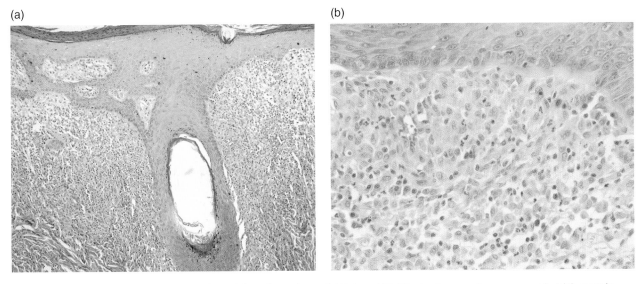

Figure 3.35 (a, b) Uveodermatologic syndrome. There is a substantial lichenoid infiltrate of macrophages, many of which contain melanin (melanophages).

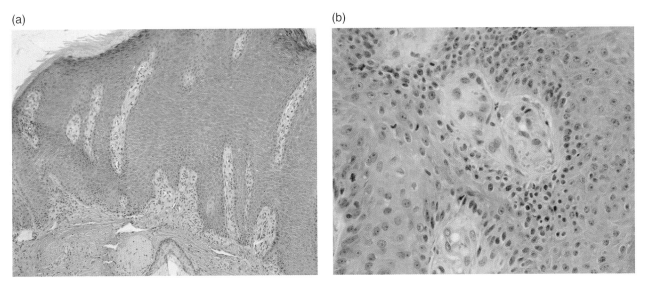

Figure 3.36 (a, b) Idiopathic equine pastern leukocytoclastic dermatitis/vasculitis. There is marked acanthosis and parakeratotic hyperkeratosis with a modest perivascular infiltrate of lymphocytes in the superficial dermis and around the deeper dermal vessels. Also, there is cell-poor to leukocytoclastic vasculitis of dermal vessels.

laminated, hyalinized walls that contain fragments of degenerate pmns, rbcs, some cell debris, and narrowed lumens, which may contain thrombi. There is frequently a modest perivascular infiltrate of lymphocytes in the superficial dermis and around the deeper dermal vessels (Figure 3.36a, b).

Bacterial Skin Disease

Bacteria of many types live on the skin but typically cause little harm. If the skin is injured by one of several other mechanisms, normal bacteriologic flora or bacterial pathogens can gain entrance to deeper layers and cause disease. The epidermis is normally a very effective barrier unless breached. Predisposing factors include things such as local or systemic viral, fungal, or parasitic infections, physical or chemical trauma, and autoimmune disease.

Pyoderma

Pyoderma literally means pus in the dermis but usually refers to purulent dermatitis caused by bacterial infection. It can be primary or secondary, superficial or deep. Mixed populations of bacteria can often be cultured from pyoderma, but Staphylococci, particularly *Staphylococcus intermedius* in dogs, are especially common causing anything from ulcerative dermatitis to folliculitis and furunculosis depending on the species of animal affected. It also causes **impetigo**, a pustular dermatitis usually of puppies.

Nocardiosis and Actinomycosis

These are bacterial infections caused by *Nocardia* sp. or *Actinomyces* sp.; there are multiple species in each genera that may cause similar lesions that can only be confirmed by culture or genetic analysis. *Nocardia* sp. are gram+, partially acid-fast filamentous bacteria that typically are found in the soil. *Actinomyces* sp. are gram+, non-acid-fast filamentous bacteria that are common within the oral cavity of many animals. Cutaneous infection is typically due to penetrating objects and results in nodular pyogranulomatous dermatitis and/or panniculitis that is ulcerated and drains to the skin surface. Organisms may be few in histopathology sections; however, substantial colonies of filamentous bacteria associated with globular aggregates of eosinophilic material (Splendore-Hoeppli reaction) may occur (Figure 3.37a–c).

Fungal Skin Disease

Dermatophytosis

Dermatophytosis is an infection of the skin and adnexa by dermatophytic fungi (*Microsporum* sp. or *Trichophyton* sp.). Lesions are limited to hairs, nails, epidermis, and dermis. These fungi prefer to grow within or upon the surface of the stratum corneum and within and on hair shafts. Microscopically the stratum corneum is thickened and contains organisms, and there is purulent to pyogranulomatous inflammation of the hair follicles with fungal hyphae and spores in hair shafts. Frequently, there is furunculosis secondary to traumatic rupture of hair follicles (Figure 3.38a, b).

Malassezia sp. are yeasts that inhabit the skin (especially ear canals) and can exacerbate some canine skin diseases. Occasionally, dermatophytes get into the dermis/subcutis and form nodules of tangled hyphae, pyogranulomatous exudate, and Splendore-Hoeppli reaction material – these are dermatophytic pseudomycetomas (Figure 3.39).

Additional Fungal Skin Disease

Other fungi can cause deeper or subcutaneous lesions, particularly granulomas or diffuse deep pyogranulomatous dermatitis, if they are introduced into the dermis by puncture wounds or if the animal is immune-compromised. *Sporothrix schenckii* is an example of this type of disease. Also, nodular aggregates of saprophytic fungi may incite formation of granulomas or pyogranulomas called mycetomas. Pigmented fungi form a subcategory, called phaeohyphomycetomas, and are especially

(a) (b) (c)

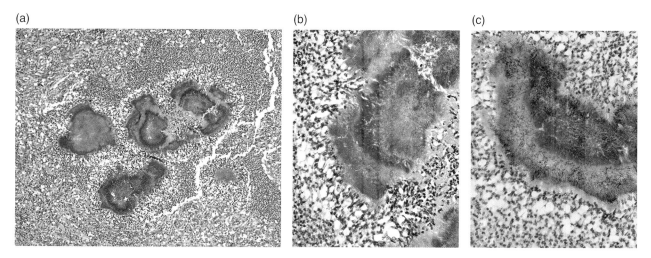

Figure 3.37   (a–c) Actinomycosis. These are colonies of gram+, non-acid-fast filamentous bacteria associated with globular aggregates of eosinophilic material (Splendore-Hoeppli reaction) and surrounded by pyogranulomatous exudate.

(a)

(b)

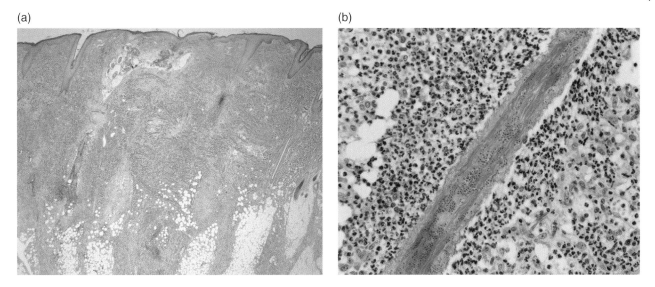

Figure 3.38 (a, b) Dermatophytosis. There is purulent to pyogranulomatous inflammation of the hair follicles with fungal hyphae and spores in hair shafts. Frequently, there is furunculosis secondary to traumatic rupture of hair follicles.

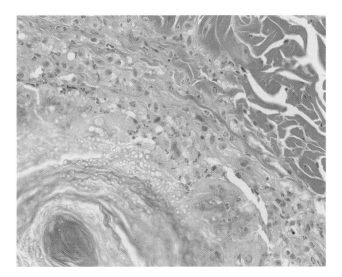

Figure 3.39 Dermatophytic pseudomycetoma. This is a nodule of tangled hyphae (hollow spaces) and pyogranulomatous exudate in the dermis and subcutis.

common in horses (Figure 3.40). Dermatitis may be a feature of the very severe systemic mycoses caused by dimorphic fungi, such as blastomycosis, histoplasmosis, and coccidioidomycosis. Cutaneous blastomycosis is caused by *Blastomyces dermatitidis*, the tissue form of which is a spherical 10–20 μm diameter yeast that has a fairly thick refractile wall and broad-based budding (Figure 3.41a, b). These organisms incite pyogranulomatous inflammation. *Cryptococcus neoformans* is a 10–15 μm diameter yeast that is surrounded by a mucinous capsule; it incites a granulomatous reaction. *Histoplasma capsulatum* is a smaller yeast form (5–8 μm in diameter) that also typically incites granulomatous inflammation.

Parasitic Skin Disease

Demodectic Mange

Many helminths and arthropods can cause various forms of dermatitis. In canine **demodicosis**, *Demodex canis* and *D. injai* primarily live in hair follicles, and when they cause disease, it is typically a transmural lymphocytic folliculitis (Figure 3.42). Trauma from scratching can result in furunculosis. *Demodex gaoti* lives in the stratum corneum and causes

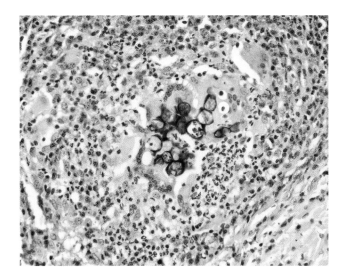

Figure 3.40 Phaeohyphomycosis. This is a nodular aggregate of saprophytic pigmented fungal hyphae surrounded by granulomatous to pyogranulomatous exudate in the dermis or subcutis.

(a)

(b)

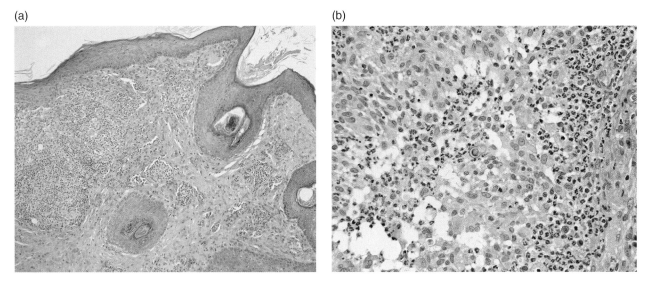

Figure 3.41 (a, b) Blastomycosis. There is multifocal pyogranulomatous exudate containing spherical 10–20 μm diameter yeasts that have a fairly thick refractile wall and broad-based budding.

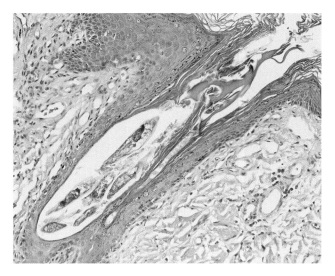

Figure 3.42 Demodectic mange. This hair follicle is filled with mites (*Demodex canis*), and there is hyperkeratosis with mild lymphoplasmacytic dermatitis.

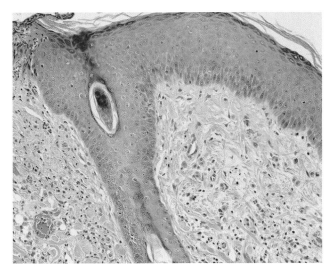

Figure 3.43   This is *Demodex gaoti* in the epidermis of a cat. There is mild to moderate superficial perivascular dermatitis.

feline superficial demodicosis, which is characterized by hyperkeratosis and acanthosis with modest superficial perivascular to diffuse dermatitis; since this condition is pruritic, there is frequently epidermal ulceration (Figure 3.43).

Sarcoptic and Notoedric Mange (Scabies)

Scabies is caused by sarcoptiform mites in dogs and cats, respectively. These mites live in the superficial epidermis and cause intense pruritus. In addition to the presence of sarcoptiform mites in and on the epidermis, characteristic lesions of scabies consist of marked hyperkeratosis with serocellular crusts, acanthosis, and moderate to marked superficial perivascular to diffuse dermatitis with eosinophils, mast cells, macrophages and scattered pmns (Figure 3.44a, b).

(a)   (b)

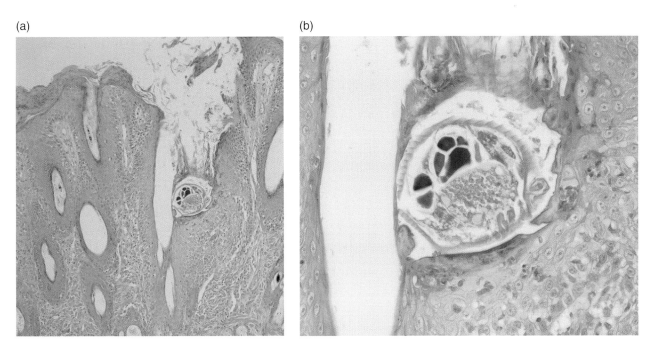

Figure 3.44   (a, b) Notoedric mange in a cat. Sarcoptiform mite (*Notoedres cati*) in the epidermis. There is hyperkeratosis, acanthosis, and superficial perivascular to diffuse dermatitis.

Cutaneous Habronemiasis

This is caused by aberrant migrating larvae of the nematodes *Habronema majus*, *H. muscae*, or *Draschia megastoma* in the skin; these larvae are transmitted by flies. The typical lesion that develops is a nodule composed of granulation tissue that contains multiple granulomas with necrotic centers with pockets of degranulated eosinophils surrounding a larval nematode (Figure 3.45a, b).

Miscellaneous Inflammatory Skin Diseases

Acral Lick Dermatitis

This is focal chronic hyperplastic dermatitis, usually on the mid- to distal limbs in dogs. There is typically marked acanthosis, hyperkeratosis, and superficial dermal fibrosis with vertical streaking of collagen (Figure 3.46).

(a) (b)

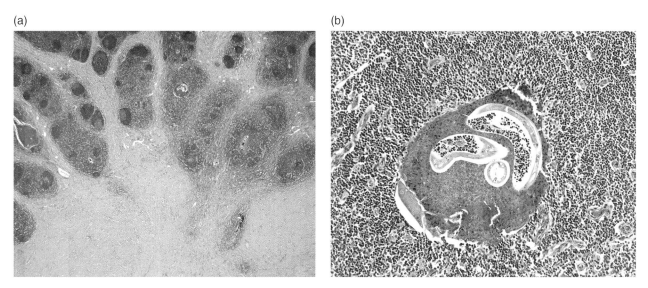

Figure 3.45   (a, b) Cutaneous habronemiasis. This lesion consists of multiple eosinophilic granulomas in the dermis, some of which contain larva of *Habronema* sp. or *Draschia megastoma*.

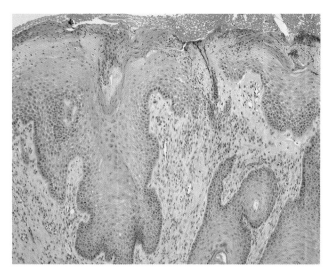

Figure 3.46   Acral lick dermatitis. This is chronic hyperplastic dermatitis characterized by marked acanthosis, hyperkeratosis, and superficial dermal fibrosis with vertical streaking of collagen.

Chronic Otitis Externa

There is typically hyperkeratosis, acanthosis with hyperplasia of sebaceous glands and cystic hyperplasia of ceruminous glands. There is a diffuse infiltrate of lymphocytes, plasma cells, pmns, and macrophages within the dermis and around the adnexae. Also, there is frequently dermal fibrosis and osseous metaplasia adjacent to the ear canal cartilage (Figure 3.47).

Pyogranulomatous Panniculitis

This is a fairly common lesion, but frequently the cause is not evident. It is characterized by a focal nodular infiltrate of macrophages, lymphocytes, plasma cells, and pmns along with fibrosis within the adipose tissue of the panniculus. Also, there frequently are pockets of pmns surrounding empty spaces, presumably where lipid had accumulated (Figure 3.48a, b).

Sebaceous Adenitis

This condition occurs in dogs and cats, with a strong canine breed predilection in the Standard Poodle, Akita, Vizula, and Samoyed. However, it occurs in many other pure bred and mixed breed dogs as well. During the active phase of the disease, there is granulomatous inflammation of the sebaceous glands and associated ducts; this results in destruction of the gland along with substantial follicular hyperkeratosis. In chronic cases, there is alopecia with follicular hyperkeratosis and complete absence of sebaceous glands with little to no remaining inflammation (Figure 3.49a–c).

Neoplasms and Cystic Lesions of the Skin

Epithelial Neoplasms

Squamous Papilloma

Papillomas (verrucae, warts) are benign, exophytic papillary neoplasms marked by proliferation of the epidermis. Most are caused by papillomaviruses, and they occur in many species. Microscopically, viral papillomas are focal lesions that are composed of fronds of proliferative stratified squamous epithelium with an appropriate pattern of differentiation aligned

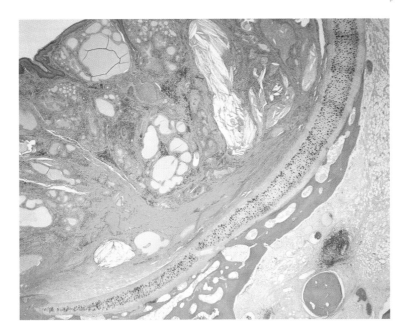

Figure 3.47   Chronic otitis externa. This is characterized by hyperkeratosis, acanthosis with hyperplasia of sebaceous glands, and cystic hyperplasia of ceruminous glands along with a diffuse infiltrate of lymphocytes, plasma cells, pmns, and macrophages. Also, there is frequently dermal fibrosis and osseous metaplasia adjacent to the ear canal cartilage.

(a)

(b)

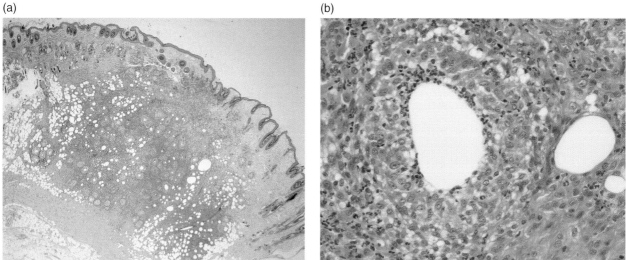

Figure 3.48 (a, b) Pyogranulomatous panniculitis. This is characterized by a focal nodular infiltrate of macrophages, lymphocytes, plasma cells, and pmns along with fibrosis within the adipose tissue of the panniculus. Also, there are frequently pockets of pmns surrounding empty spaces, presumably where lipid had accumulated.

(a)

(b)

(c)

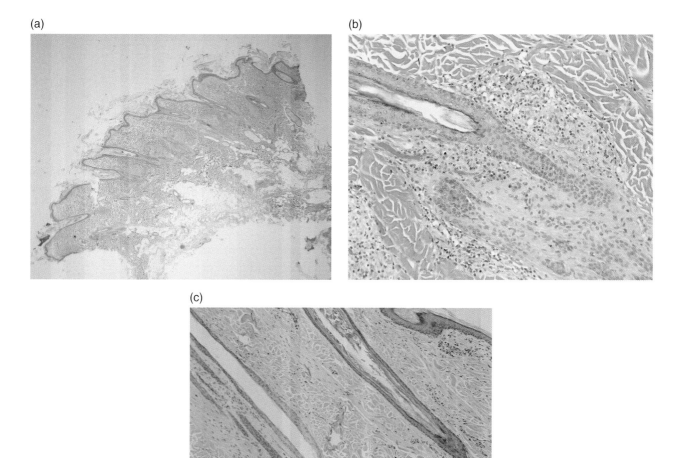

Figure 3.49 (a, b) Sebaceous adenitis. This is granulomatous inflammation of the sebaceous glands and associated ducts, which results in destruction of the gland along with substantial follicular hyperkeratosis. (c) This is chronic sebaceous adenitis, in which destruction of the gland has resulted in complete absence of sebaceous glands with little to no remaining inflammation.

(a) (b)

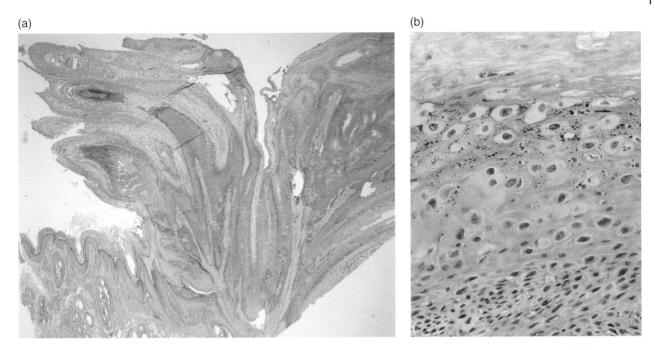

Figure 3.50 (a, b) Squamous papilloma due to canine papillomavirus. This is composed of fronds of proliferative stratified squamous epithelium aligned upon a fibrovascular core. The stratum corneum is thickened, and the stratum granulosum contains cells containing prominent keratohyaline granules and vacuolated epidermal cells that have a somewhat condensed nucleus (koilocytes). Occasional epidermal cells contain a vague intranuclear eosinophilic viral inclusion body.

upon a fibrovascular core. The stratum corneum is somewhat thickened. The stratum granulosum is also thickened and many cells contain prominent keratohyalin granules; some cells contain a vague eosinophilic intranuclear viral inclusion body. Also, there are vacuolated epidermal cells that have a somewhat condensed nucleus; these are koilocytes (Figure 3.50a, b). It is common to have a moderate dermal infiltrate of lymphocytes and plasma cells subjacent to the mass, especially late in its course. Nonviral squamous papillomas also occur and have a similar appearance, but lack intranuclear viral inclusion bodies and koilocytes.

Inverted Viral Squamous Papilloma
Inverted viral squamous papillomas occur in dogs and are also caused by a papillomavirus. These are composed of a focal area of proliferative epidermis that invaginates into the dermis, below the level of the adjacent epidermis. The cytologic changes in the epidermal cells are similar to those of exophytic viral papillomas (Figure 3.51a, b).

Cutaneous Horn
Cutaneous horns are benign, horn-shaped masses of keratin that project above the skin; they may be single or multiple (Figure 3.52a, b).

Canine and Feline Viral Plaque
Canine and Feline Viral plaques are caused by papillomaviruses and are composed of focal plaques of proliferative epidermis that have somewhat prominent scalloped rete ridges. Epidermal cells typically contain prominent keratohyaline granules, and occasionally koilocytes are evident (Figure 3.53a, b). Also, some canine viral plaques are pigmented (Figure 3.53c, d).

Actinic Keratosis
Actinic keratosis is a proliferative epidermal lesion that occurs in areas of little to no pigmentation and is caused by epidermal injury from ultraviolet radiation. It is a plaque-like lesion that is hyperkeratotic and has cytologic abnormalities that range from epidermal dysplasia to in situ squamous cell carcinoma.

(a) 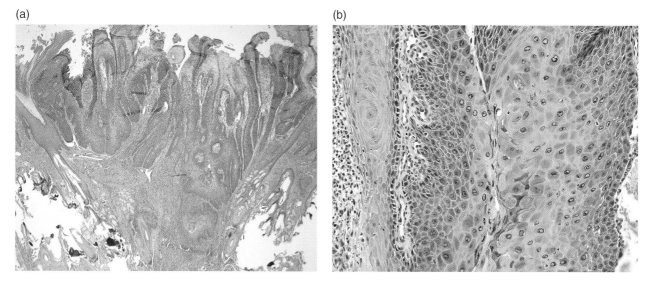 (b)

Figure 3.51   (a, b) Inverted viral squamous papilloma. The proliferative stratified squamous epithelium invaginates into the dermis. The cytologic changes in the epidermal cells are similar to those of exophytic viral papillomas.

(a) 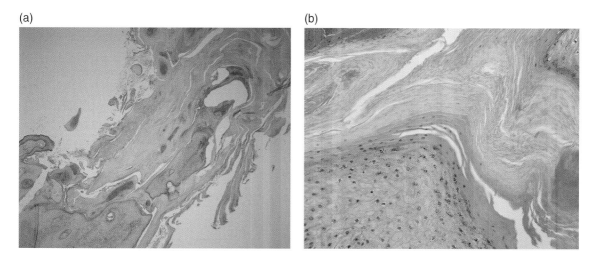 (b)

Figure 3.52   (a, b) Cutaneous horn. This is a horn-shaped mass of dense, laminated keratin that projects above the underlying proliferative stratified squamous epithelium.

Squamous Cell Carcinoma

Squamous cell carcinoma (SCC) is a malignant neoplasm of stratified squamous cells of the epidermis and mucous membranes. Grossly, they usually begin as gray or depigmented nodules with a crusty surface that may proliferate upward and become ulcerated or may send long, irregular, penetrating cords of neoplastic cells into the dermis and subcutis. This infiltrative form may become ulcerated superficially and appear as a crater. Cutaneous SCC may occur in a variety of locations, but especially around the eyes, ears, face, and toes. Nonpigmented skin is at risk of SCC due to injury from ultraviolet radiation, and several forms of SCC are known to develop from premalignant proliferative lesions caused by papilloma viruses. A variety of patterns exist ranging from in situ SCC to invasive SCC. Microscopically, neoplastic cells can vary from polygonal to spindle, with little to marked pleomorphism; desmosomes may be evident in some areas. In situ, SCC is a focal proliferative epidermal lesion characterized by some degree of pleomorphism, lack of normal polarity, and increased mitotic rate but is still confined by the epidermal basement membrane. Bowenoid in situ SCC is a multifocal lesion that most frequently occurs in cats and is associated with feline papillomavirus infection. Neoplastic cells in invasive SCC typically form a sheet, frequently with round masses of laminated keratin, which may have acantholytic centers that contain

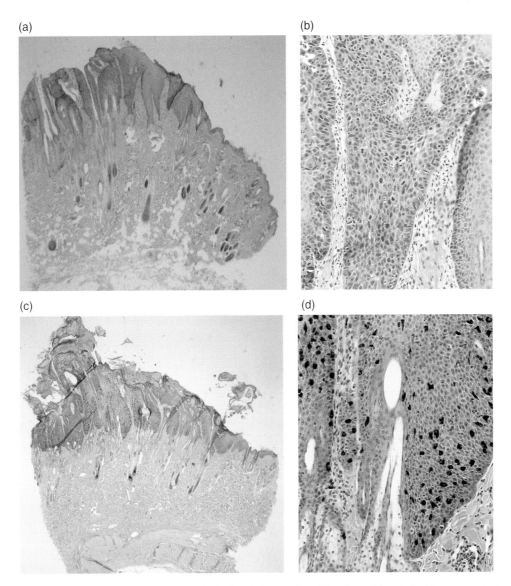

Figure 3.53 (a, b) Feline viral plaque. This is composed of a focal plaque of proliferative epidermis that has somewhat prominent scalloped rete ridges. Epidermal cells typically contain prominent keratohyaline granules, and occasionally koilocytes. (c, d) Canine pigmented viral plaque. This is composed of a focal plaque of proliferative epidermis that has somewhat prominent scalloped rete ridges and melanin-containing cells.

pmns. Invasive SCC is characterized by invasive finger-like projections into the adjacent dermis and/or lymphatics that usually incite desmoplasia, which is the proliferation of non-neoplastic immature fibrovascular tissue.

Squamous Cell Carcinoma
In situ canine (Figure 3.54a, b)
In situ feline (Figure 3.55a, b)
Bowenoid (Figure 3.56a, b)
Spindle cell (Figure 3.57)
Acantholytic (Figure 3.58a, b)
Canine subungual (Figure 3.59)
Feline (Figure 3.60)
Equine (Figure 3.61a, b)

(a)

(b)

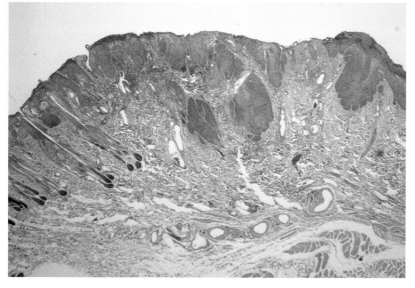
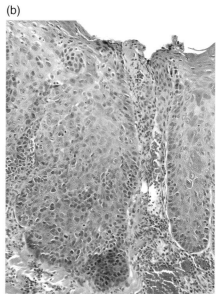

Figure 3.54   (a, b) Canine in situ squamous cell carcinoma.

(a)

(b)

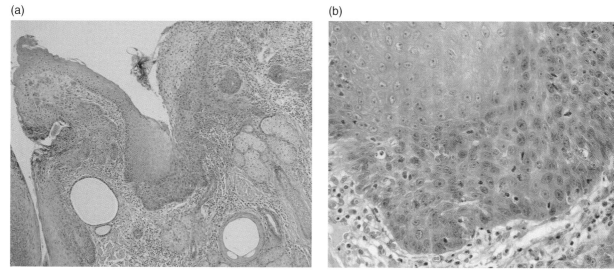

Figure 3.55   (a, b) Feline in situ squamous cell carcinoma.

(a)

(b)

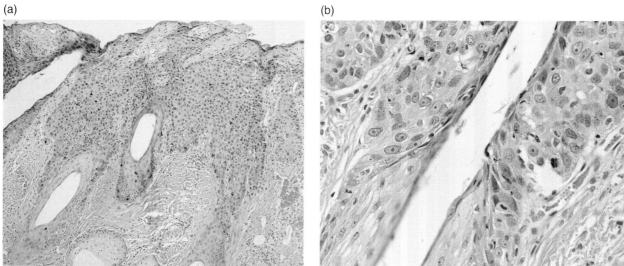

Figure 3.56   (a, b) Bowenoid squamous cell carcinoma in situ in a cat.

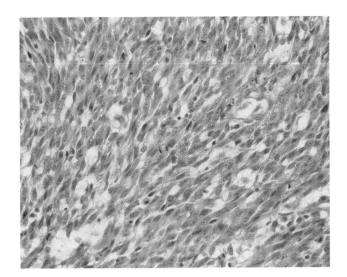

Figure 3.57   Spindle cell squamous cell carcinoma.

(a)

(b)

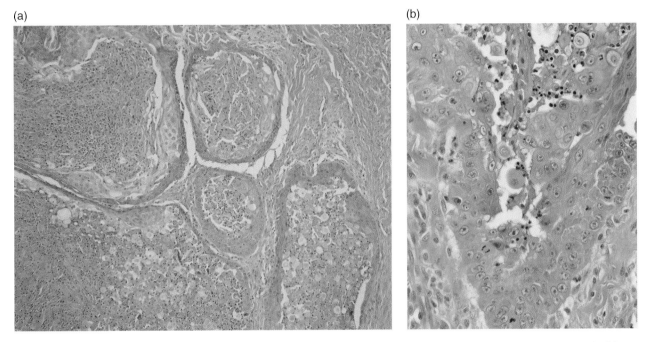

Figure 3.58   (a, b) Acantholytic squamous cell carcinoma. Neoplastic keratinocytes in the center of these lobules have detached from one another. The acantholytic centers also frequently contain pmns.

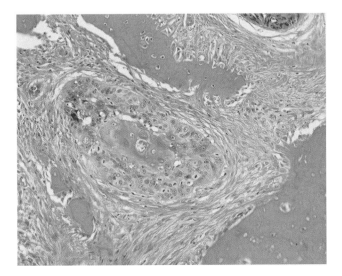

Figure 3.59   Canine subungual squamous cell carcinoma.

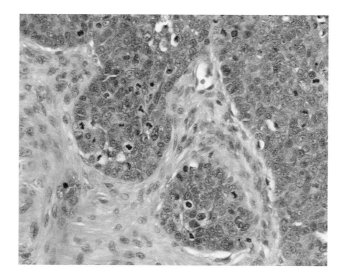

Figure 3.60   Feline squamous cell carcinoma. There is an invasion of the dermis by finger, like projections of neoplastic cells, which have incited desmoplasia.

(a)   (b)

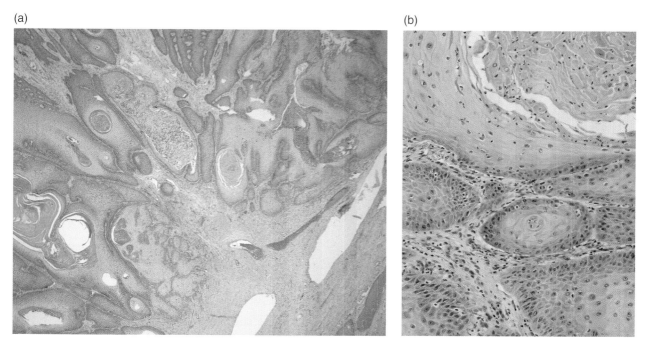

Figure 3.61   (a, b) Equine squamous cell carcinoma. This is a well-differentiated squamous cell carcinoma. There are numerous "keratin pearls" along with finger-like projections of neoplastic cells into the adjacent dermis.

Basosquamous Carcinoma

Basosquamous carcinoma is an invasive neoplasm composed of basaloid cells, which are relatively small and dark, and squamous cells, which are larger, polygonal, and resemble those in SCC. There is a fairly abrupt transition between these two neoplastic cell populations (Figure 3.62a, b).

Infundibular Keratinizing Acanthoma (Intracutaneous Cornifying Epithelioma)

Infundibular keratinizing acanthoma is a benign neoplasm that has differentiation toward the infundibular portion of the hair follicle. It is characterized by an invaginated, circumscribed mass that is composed of a peripheral rim of well-differentiated stratified squamous epithelium and a cystic center that is typically filled with laminated keratin and opens

(a)

(b)

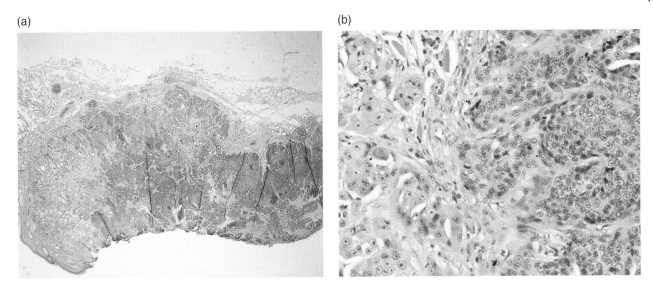

Figure 3.62 (a, b) Basosquamous carcinoma in a cat. This is a plaque-like mass composed of neoplastic basal cells along with squamous differentiation.

to the epidermal surface through a pore. These are frequently traumatized, which results in discharge of keratin into the adjacent dermis, inciting granulomatous to pyogranulomatous dermatitis (Figure 3.63a, b).

Subungual Keratoacanthoma

Subungual keratoacanthoma is a benign neoplasm arising in the nailbed epithelium. It is composed of a circumscribed mass of well-differentiated stratified squamous epithelium, frequently with a cystic center filled with laminated keratin, somewhat resembling an infundibular keratinizing acanthoma or an inverted viral papilloma. As it expands, it will stimulate lysis of P3, and if traumatized and ruptured, will incite granulomatous to pyogranulomatous inflammation (Figure 3.64).

Trichoblastoma (Basal Cell Tumor)

Trichoblastoma is a benign neoplasm derived from the stratum basale of the epidermis. The basal cells lack the desmosomes (intercellular bridges) of the stratum spinosum, that occur in squamous cell carcinomas and papillomas. The neoplastic cells are relatively small and have an oval hyperchromatic nucleus and a modest amount of eosinophilic cytoplasm. Trichoblastomas are typically circumscribed, thinly encapsulated masses that may have one of several microscopic patterns. Occasionally, there is malignant transformation to **malignant trichoblastoma**, which is frequently ulcerated and incites desmoplasia as it invades into the adjacent dermis.

Trichoblastoma

Solid (Figure 3.65)
Glandular (Figure 3.66)
Cystic (Figure 3.67a, b)
Lobular (Figure 3.68a, b)
Medusoid (Figure 3.69)
Ribbon (Figure 3.70)
Feline pigmented (Figure 3.71a, b)

Trichoepithelioma

Trichoepithelioma is a multilobular plaque-like neoplasm, each lobule of which contains one or more segments of hair follicle development (Figure 3.72). Lobules typically have a combination of basilar and stratified squamous epithelium surrounding a central laminated aggregate of keratin, which sometimes resembles a hair shaft (Figure 3.73a). This neoplasm is typically benign but occasionally becomes invasive into the adjacent dermis, which would be considered a **malignant trichoepithelioma** (Figure 3.73b).

(a)

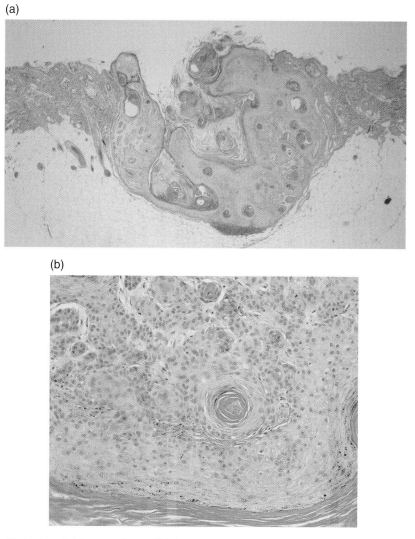

(b)

Figure 3.63 (a, b) Infundibular keratinizing acanthoma. This is a cup-shaped, invaginated mass of well-differentiated stratified squamous epithelium with a cystic center that is filled with laminated keratin and opens to the epidermal surface by a pore.

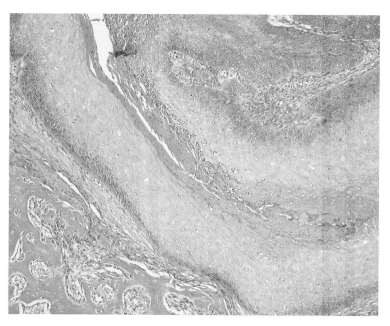

Figure 3.64 Subungual keratoacanthoma.

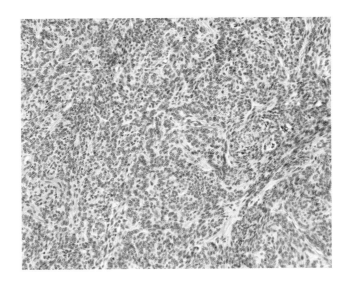

Figure 3.65   Trichoblastoma, solid pattern.

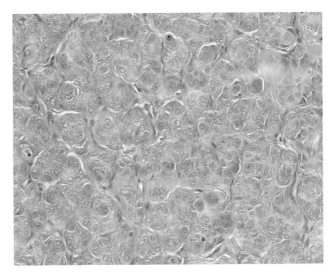

Figure 3.66   Trichoblastoma, glandular pattern.

(a)

(b)

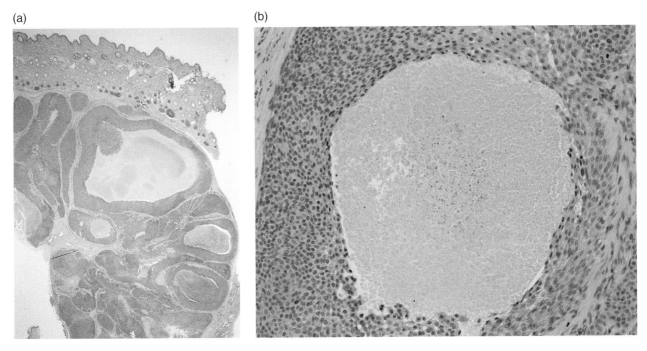

Figure 3.67   (a, b) Trichoblastoma, cystic.

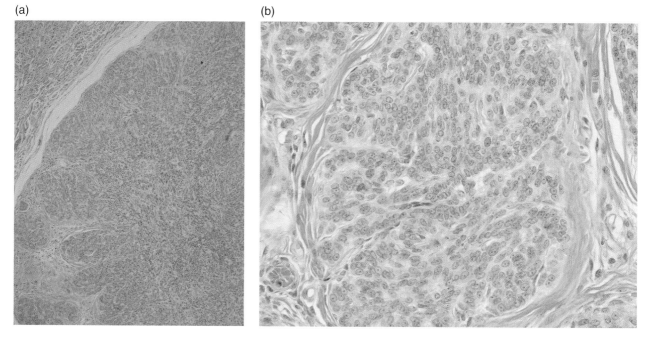

Figure 3.68 (a, b) Trichoblastoma, lobular pattern.

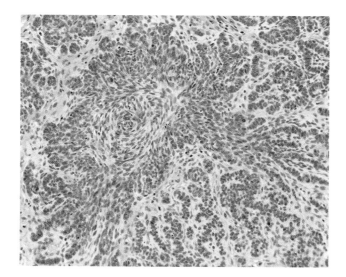

Figure 3.69 Trichoblastoma, Medusoid pattern.

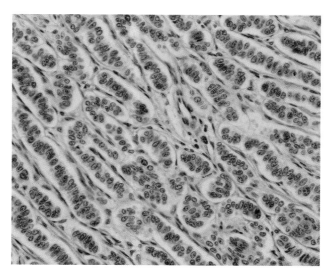

Figure 3.70 Trichoblastoma, ribbon pattern.

(a)

(b)

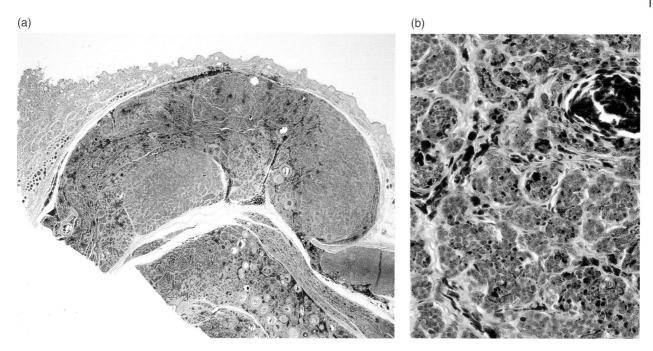

Figure 3.71   (a, b) Feline pigmented trichoblastoma.

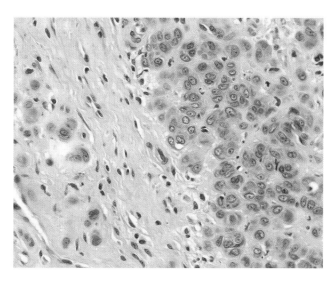

Figure 3.72   Malignant trichoblastoma in a dog. Neoplastic basaloid cells are aligned in small aggregates and lobules, some of which have invaded the adjacent fibrous stroma.

Pilomatricoma

Pilomatricoma is a multilobular neoplasm that has differentiation toward hair follicle development. Each lobule is typically composed of a peripheral zone of basilar epithelium with abrupt transition to a central sheet of keratinized epithelium ("ghost cells") that resemble hair matrix. These ghost cells are polygonal and have abundant eosinophilic cytoplasm and a central lucent area in place of a nucleus. In many cases, this keratinized central area is pigmented due to melanin, and/or mineralized; occasionally, there is osseous metaplasia in the center of these lobules (Figure 3.74a, b). This neoplasm is typically benign but occasionally becomes invasive into the adjacent dermis, which would be considered a **malignant pilomatricoma**.

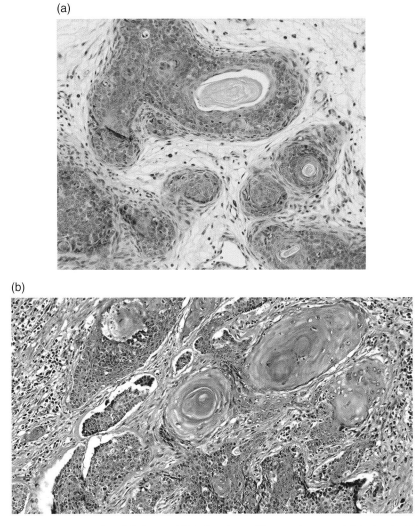

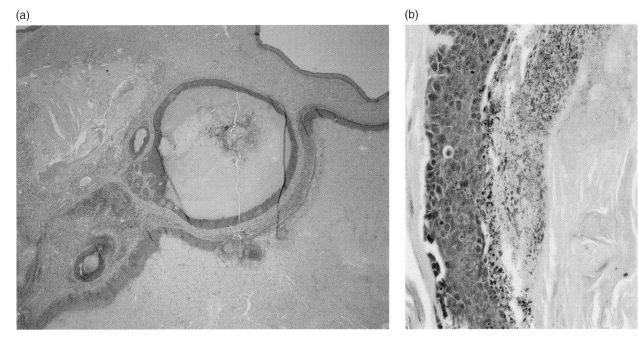

Figure 3.73   (a) Trichoepithelioma from a dog. This is a multilobular plaque-like neoplasm, each lobule of which contains one or more segments of hair follicle development. (b) Malignant trichoepithelioma from a dog. The mitotic index is high, and the neoplastic tissue is more invasive than the typical trichoepithelioma and incites desmoplasia.

Figure 3.74   (a, b) Pilomatricoma.

Apocrine Gland Tumors

Apocrine gland tumors range from adenoma to adenocarcinoma. **Adenomas** are multilobular neoplasms that are composed of tubuloacinar structures lined by a single layer of well-differentiated cuboidal epithelial cells that have a dome-shaped luminal surface; occasionally, there may be decapitation buds along the luminal surface of cells, consistent with apocrine secretion. Some variants have cystic dilation of acini, forming an **apocrine cystadenoma** (Figure 3.75); occasionally, there are papillary fronds of epithelium within the cystic lumens. Neoplasms may also arise within the apocrine gland ducts (**apocrine ductular adenoma**) (Figure 3.76a, b); these are characterized by a double layer of cuboidal epithelium forming ductular structures. Local invasion into the dermis is indicative of malignant behavior (**apocrine adenocarcinoma**) (Figure 3.77a, b).

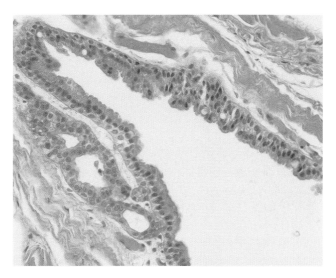

Figure 3.75   Apocrine gland cystadenoma. This is composed of tubuloacinar structures lined by a single layer of well-differentiated cuboidal epithelial cells that have a dome-shaped luminal surface. Occasionally there are papillary fronds of epithelium within the cystic lumens.

(a)   (b)

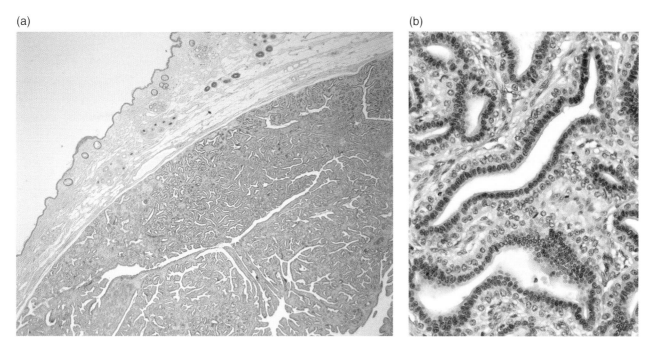

Figure 3.76   (a, b) Apocrine ductular adenoma. This is composed of tubuloacinar structures lined by a double layer of well-differentiated cuboidal epithelial cells.

(a) (b)

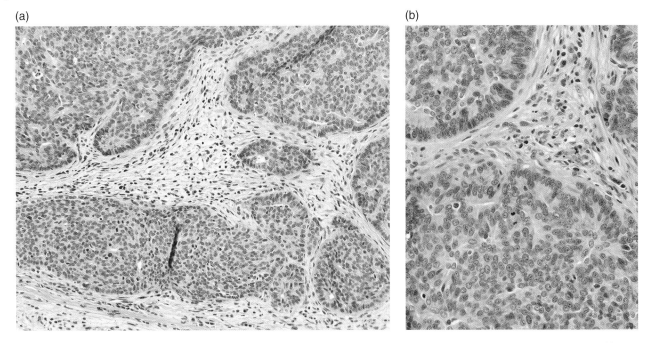

Figure 3.77   (a, b) Apocrine adenocarcinoma. These are invasive, multilobular neoplasms that are composed of cuboidal epithelium with a moderate amount of eosinophilic cytoplasm and an oval hyperchromatic nucleus.

Anal Sac Apocrine Adenocarcinoma

Anal sac apocrine adenocarcinoma is a somewhat unique version of an apocrine gland adenocarcinoma that arises from the apocrine glands of the anal sac in dogs. These have a different microscopic appearance than cutaneous apocrine adenocarcinomas, and may resemble neuroendocrine neoplasms. They are invasive, multilobular neoplasms that are composed of cuboidal epithelium with a moderate amount of eosinophilic cytoplasm and an oval hyperchromatic nucleus aligned in palisading rows along a fine fibrovascular stroma. There are occasional acinar structures and pseudorosettes scattered throughout the neoplasm (Figure 3.78a, b). These neoplasms are noted for causing the paraneoplastic syndrome of hypercalcemia due to the secretion of parathyroid hormone-related peptide.

(a) (b)

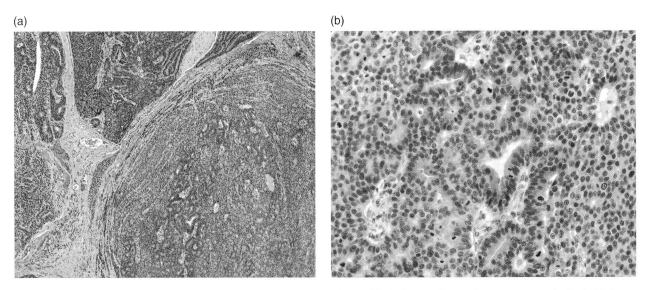

Figure 3.78   (a, b) Anal sac apocrine adenocarcinoma. These are invasive, multilobular neoplasms that are composed of cuboidal epithelium with a moderate amount of eosinophilic cytoplasm and an oval hyperchromatic nucleus aligned in palisading rows along a fine fibrovascular stroma with occasional acinar structures and pseudorosettes.

Ceruminous Gland Tumors

Ceruminous gland tumors are derived from the ceruminous glands of the external ear canal. **Adenomas** are composed of cuboidal to columnar cells that have a single oval nucleus, 1–2 prominent nucleoli, a moderate amount of eosinophilic cytoplasm, and discernible cell borders. Anisocytosis and anisokaryosis are minimal, and the mitotic rate is low. The lumens of the glands may be cystic and contain papillary projections (Figure 3.79a, b). Also, **adenocarcinomas** occur, and these are characterized by invasive behavior that incites desmoplasia (Figure 3.80).

Sebaceous Gland Tumors

Sebaceous gland tumors are categorized as either focal or multifocal sebaceous gland hyperplasia, adenoma, epithelioma, or carcinoma. **Focal/multifocal sebaceous hyperplasia** is a common cutaneous lesion is older dogs and is composed of proliferative, well-differentiated sebaceous glands surrounding a duct lined by stratified squamous epithelium (Figure 3.81a, b).

(a)   (b)

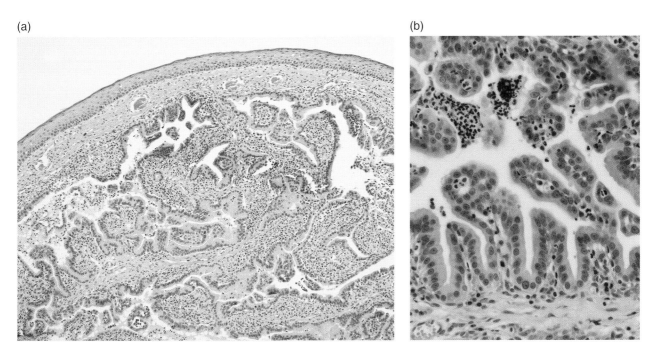

Figure 3.79   (a, b) Ceruminous gland cystadenoma.

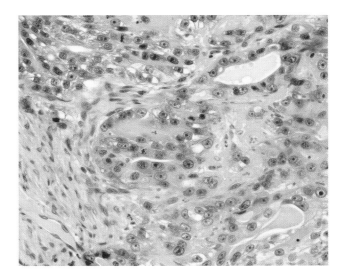

Figure 3.80   Ceruminous gland adenocarcinoma.

(a)

(b)

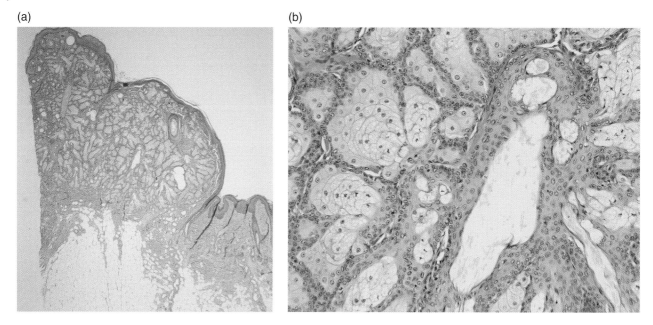

Figure 3.81   (a, b) Focal sebaceous hyperplasia.

Adenomas are composed of multiple lobules of well-differentiated sebocytes along with a larger number of basal cells and are less organized (Figure 3.82a, b). **Sebaceous epitheliomas** are multilobular masses within the dermis that are composed of proliferative basal cells with a few differentiated sebocytes and small, keratinized ductules, and frequently have a cavitated center filled with cell debris; the mitotic index is moderate to high (Figure 3.83). **Sebaceous carcinomas** are invasive, incite desmoplasia and are composed of multiple lobules of neoplastic polyhedral cells, some of which contain lipid vacuoles; these typically have a moderate to high mitotic index (Figure 3.84).

(a)

(b)

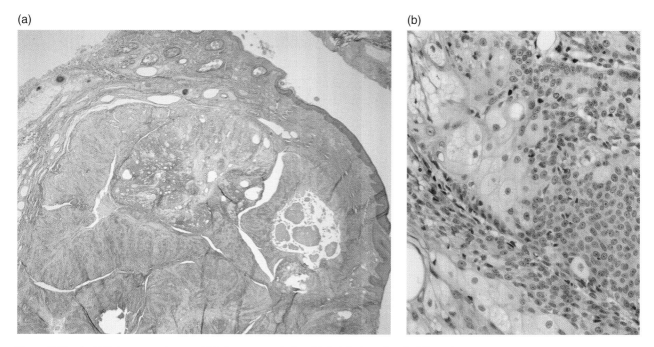

Figure 3.82   (a, b) Sebaceous adenoma. This is composed of multiple lobules of well-differentiated sebocytes along with a larger number of basal cells.

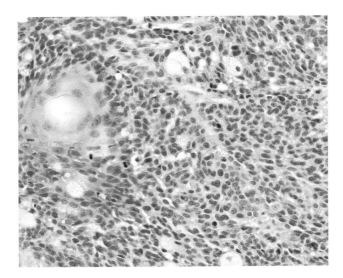

Figure 3.83 Sebaceous epithelioma. These are multilobular masses that are composed of proliferative basal cells with a few differentiated sebocytes and small, keratinized ductules.

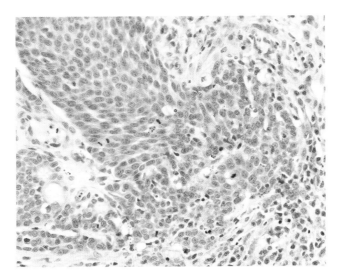

Figure 3.84 Sebaceous carcinoma. These are composed of multiple lobules of neoplastic polyhedral to spindle cells with a moderate to high mitotic index, some of which may contain lipid vacuoles.

Hepatoid/Perianal Gland Tumors

Hepatoid/Perianal gland tumors occur most commonly in old male dogs but also occur in spayed female dogs. They occur around the anus, at the base of the tail, and at the preputial orifice. These neoplasms are composed of discrete lobules, each with a central aggregate of large polygonal cells with abundant eosinophilic cytoplasm, distinct cell borders, and a peripheral rim of small cuboidal reserve cells. **Adenomas**, which are much more common than malignant tumors, have a low mitotic index and are well-differentiated (Figure 3.85a, b). **Carcinomas** have a higher mitotic index, are less differentiated and are hypercellular with a higher percentage of reserve cells (Figure 3.86).

Eccrine Gland Tumors

Eccrine glands are a type of sweat gland that are present in the feet of dogs. They are tubuloacinar glands that are composed of a single layer of cuboidal epithelium. Occasionally they develop neoplasms, either eccrine adenoma or adenocarcinoma (Figure 3.87a, b).

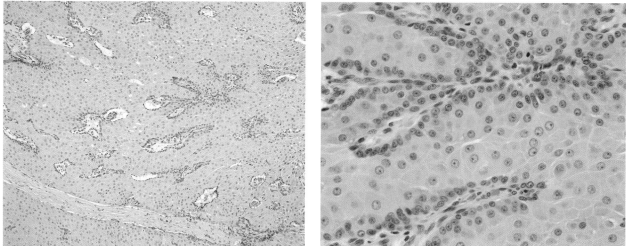

Figure 3.85 (a, b) Hepatoid/perianal gland adenoma. These neoplasms are composed of discrete lobules, each with a central aggregate of large polygonal cells with abundant eosinophilic cytoplasm, distinct cell borders, and a peripheral rim of small cuboidal reserve cells.

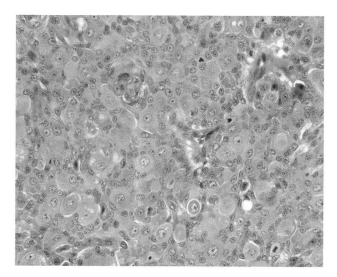

Figure 3.86 Hepatoid/perianal gland adenocarcinoma. Compared to adenomas, adenocarcinomas have a less defined lobular structure, and have a higher mitotic index, are less differentiated, and are hypercellular with a higher percentage of reserve cells.

(a)

(b)

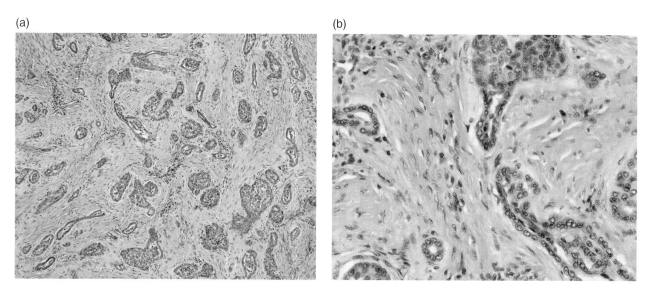

Figure 3.87 (a, b) Eccrine gland adenocarcinoma. These are composed of invasive tubuloacinar structures lined by cuboidal epithelial cells surrounded by fibrous tissue.

Melanotic Tumors

Melanotic tumors are common skin neoplasms in dogs and horses but less common in cats. Malignancy in dogs depends mostly on location. Those on the eyelid and trunk (less than 1 cm) are generally benign, while those in the oral cavity, on the digits, on the scrotum, and those greater than 2 cm on the trunk are typically malignant. Melanomas are fairly common in the perineal/perianal area and under the tail of gray horses. Microscopically, benign tumors (**melanocytomas**) are typically discrete, heavily pigmented masses composed of moderate to large, round to spindle cells that contain numerous melanosomes; these have a low mitotic index and minimal to moderate anisocytosis and anisokaryosis (Figure 3.88). **Malignant melanomas** are typically invasive and are composed of round to spindle cells with discernible cell borders, aligned in sheets and packets. Malignant melanocytes usually have a high mitotic index, moderate to marked anisocytosis and anisokaryosis, and a minimal to substantial amount of cytoplasmic melanin. Malignant melanocytes will frequently invade the adjacent epithelium (junctional activity) (Figure 3.89). Also, malignant melanomas may metastasize, especially to the lungs and regional lymph nodes.

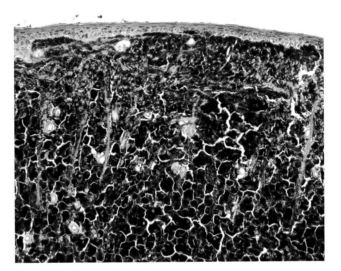

Figure 3.88 Melanocytoma. These are composed of moderate to large, round to spindle cells that contain numerous melanosomes, have a low mitotic index and minimal to moderate anisocytosis and anisokaryosis.

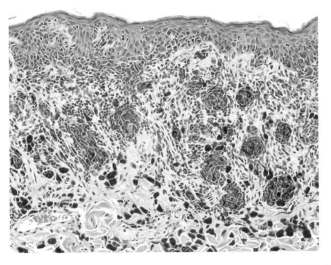

Figure 3.89 Malignant melanoma. These are invasive and composed of round to spindle cells with discernible cell borders that are aligned in sheets and packets. Malignant melanocytes usually have a high mitotic index, moderate to marked anisocytosis and anisokaryosis, and a minimal to substantial amount of cytoplasmic melanin. Malignant melanocytes will frequently invade the adjacent epithelium (junctional activity).

Canine Soft Tissue Sarcomas

Many canine sarcomas of the skin and subjacent soft tissues are included in the category of soft tissue sarcoma, grades I–III. Grading criteria are composed of the degree of differentiation, mitotic index, and amount of necrosis. Grade I sarcomas have a low mitotic index, are well differentiated, and lack necrosis, whereas grade III sarcomas have a high mitotic index, are poorly differentiated, and contain multiple foci of necrosis (Figure 3.90a–d). Soft tissue sarcomas include fibrosarcoma, vascular wall tumor (hemangiopericytoma), and peripheral neve sheath tumor.

Fibrosarcoma   This is typically an invasive mass that is composed of intersecting bundles of spindle cells that have an oval nucleus, 1–2 nucleoli, a moderate amount of eosinophilic cytoplasm and somewhat indistinct cell borders, separated by a variable amount of collagen (Figure 3.91a, b).

Vascular Wall Tumor (Hemangiopericytoma)   This is a very common cutaneous tumor in dogs but is rare in other animals. These are somewhat circumscribed, multilobular tumors that are partially encapsulated. Microscopically they are composed of spindle-shaped cells that have an oval nucleus, 1–2 nucleoli, a moderate amount of eosinophilic cytoplasm and somewhat indistinct cell borders aligned in palisades, bundles, and/or whorls of concentric rings around small vessels (Figure 3.92a–d). They rarely metastasize but will regrow if incompletely removed.

(a)

(b)

(c)

(d)

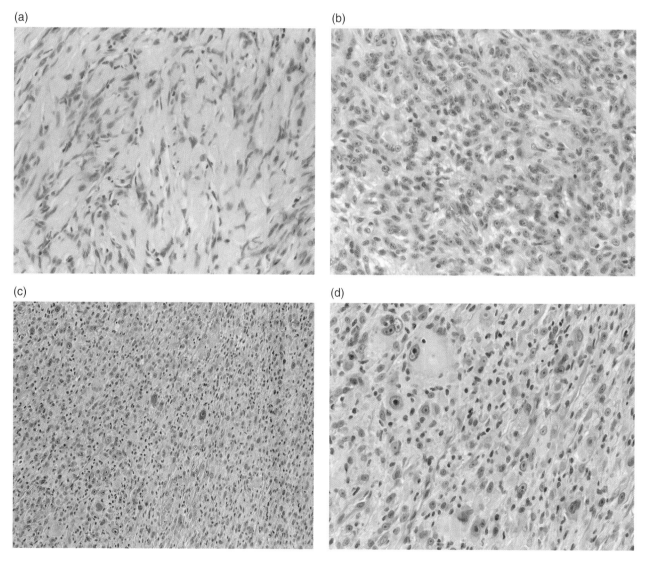

Figure 3.90   (a) Soft tissue sarcoma, grade I. (b) Soft tissue sarcoma, grade II. (c, d) Soft tissue sarcoma, grade III.

(a)

(b)

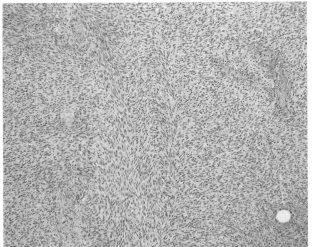

Figure 3.91　(a, b) Fibrosarcoma, grade II.

(a)

(b)

(c)

(d)

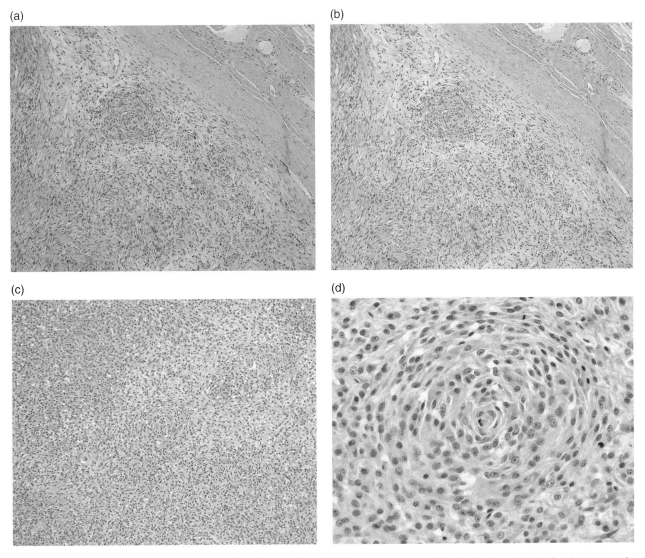

Figure 3.92　(a, b) Vascular wall tumor (hemangiopericytoma) grade I. These are composed of spindle-shaped cells that have an oval nucleus, 1–2 nucleoli, a moderate amount of eosinophilic cytoplasm, and somewhat indistinct cell borders aligned in palisades, bundles, and/or whorls of concentric rings around small vessels. (c, d) Vascular wall tumor (hemangiopericytoma), grade II.

Peripheral Nerve Sheath Tumors (Schwannoma) These are common cutaneous neoplasms, especially in dogs. Grossly and microscopically, they resemble vascular wall tumors, except palisading of neoplastic cells is more pronounced in PNSTs, and they generally lack perivascular whorls of neoplastic cells (Figure 3.93a, b).

Equine Sarcoid

Equine sarcoid is a fibroblastic neoplasm caused by infection with bovine papillomavirus types 1 or 2 in horses. These are typically broad-based growths with an irregular surface. They occur most commonly at the base of the ear, on the neck, and on limbs. They are located in the dermis and are composed of proliferative epidermis that extends rete pegs deep into a sheet of spindle cells that are aligned in intersecting bundles or palisades and separated by collagen (Figure 3.94a, b). The overlying epidermis is often ulcerated. Often multiple, they tend to recur following excision but do not metastasize.

(a)

(b)

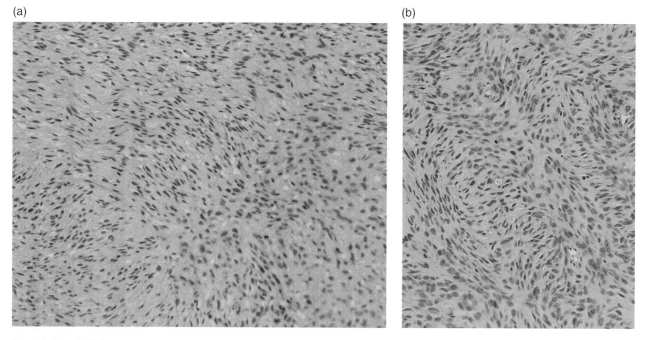

Figure 3.93   (a, b) Peripheral nerve sheath tumor, grade I.

(a)

(b)

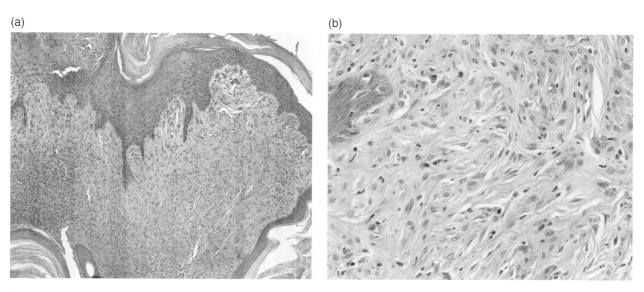

Figure 3.94   (a, b) Equine sarcoid. These are composed of proliferative epidermis that extends rete pegs deep into a sheet of spindle cells that are aligned in intersecting bundles or palisades and separated by collagen.

(a)

(b)

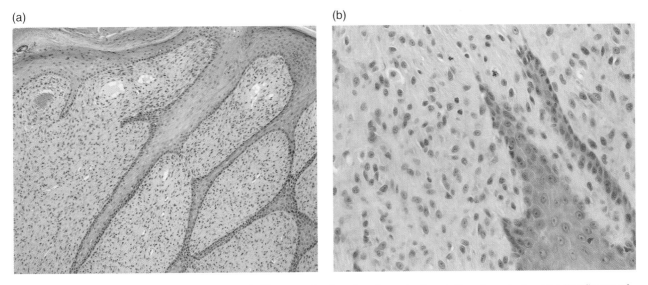

Figure 3.95 (a, b) Feline sarcoid. This is composed of interweaving bundles of neoplastic spindle cells and a few invading fingers of proliferative stratified squamous epithelium in the dermis. The neoplastic cells have a central oval to elongate nucleus, 1–2 nucleoli, a moderate amount of eosinophilic cytoplasm, and indistinct cell borders.

Feline Sarcoid

Feline sarcoid is a low-grade sarcoma that is considered to be similar to the equine sarcoid and is apparently caused by infection with papillomavirus. Feline sarcoid is a locally invasive neoplasm that does not metastasize but may return following incomplete surgical clearance. Microscopically, feline sarcoid is composed of interweaving bundles of neoplastic spindle cells and a few invading fingers of proliferative stratified squamous epithelium in the dermis. The neoplastic cells have a central oval to elongate nucleus, 1–2 nucleoli, a moderate amount of eosinophilic cytoplasm and indistinct cell borders (Figure 3.95a, b). They may spontaneously regress and the long-term prognosis is fair to good once complete clearance is achieved.

Canine Keloidal Fibroma

Canine keloidal fibroma is a benign fibrous neoplasm that is a circumscribed, nonencapsulated, plaque-like mass in the dermis that typically extends down to the cutaneous muscle. It is composed of bundles of well-differentiated fibrocytes and dense collagen, with a few scattered macrophages and mast cells. In the center, there are prominent hyalinized bundles of collagen bordered by laminated spindle cells. The mitotic index is low (<1 mitosis/10 400× fields) (Figure 3.96a, b).

Feline Giant Cell Sarcoma

Feline giant cell sarcoma is a recognized form of cutaneous sarcoma in cats that usually occurs on the extremities. Microscopically, these are an invasive mass in the dermis and subcutis that is composed of interweaving bundles of spindle cells, large round to polyhedral cells, and multinucleate giant cells. The spindle cells have an oval nucleus, 1–2 small nucleoli, a moderate amount of eosinophilic fibrillar cytoplasm, and indistinct cell borders. The giant cells have 3–5 round nuclei, abundant eosinophilic cytoplasm, and ragged cell borders. The mitotic index is typically high (Figure 3.97a, b).

Feline Vaccination Site Sarcoma

Cats may develop a sarcoma at the site of vaccination. The histomorphology of these sarcomas may vary but is usually an aggressive fibrosarcoma. There is typically a peripheral zone that contains a multifocal infiltrate of lymphocytes and scattered macrophages, which sometimes contain pale basophilic intracytoplasmic material (Figure 3.98a, b).

Cutaneous Hemangioma and Hemangiosarcoma

Cavernous Hemangioma   This is a circumscribed benign cutaneous neoplasm that is composed of substantial vascular spaces lined by a single layer of normal-appearing endothelium. The vascular spaces are typically filled with blood and occasionally contain thrombi (Figure 3.99a).

(a)

(b)

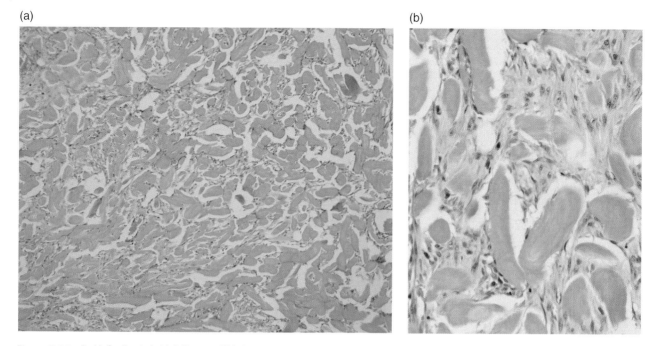

Figure 3.96   (a, b) Canine keloidal fibroma. This is composed of bundles of well-differentiated fibrocytes and dense collagen, with a few scattered macrophages and mast cells. In the center, there are prominent hyalinized bundles of collagen bordered by laminated spindle cells.

(a)

(b)

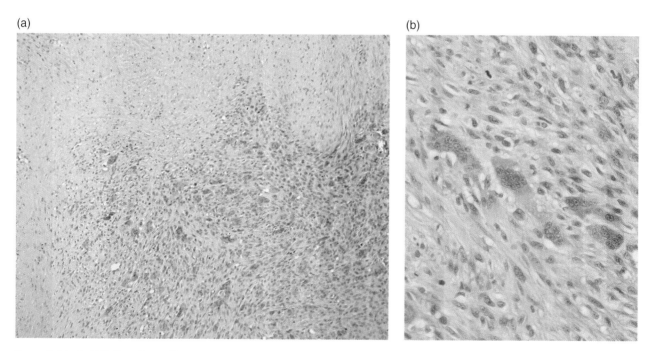

Figure 3.97   (a, b) Feline giant cell sarcoma.

Granulation Tissue Type Hemangioma   This is a type of cutaneous hemangioma that has an unusual microscopic pattern. This pattern lacks substantial vascular spaces but instead is composed of spindle cells, some of which are forming small indistinct spaces filled with blood. The neoplastic cells have an oval nucleus, 1–2 nucleoli, a moderate amount of eosinophilic cytoplasm, and an indistinct cell border. These small vascular spaces are separated by loose fibrous tissue that contains a modest infiltrate of lymphocytes, plasma cells, and mast cells. The mitotic index is low (Figure 3.99b, c).

(a)

(b)

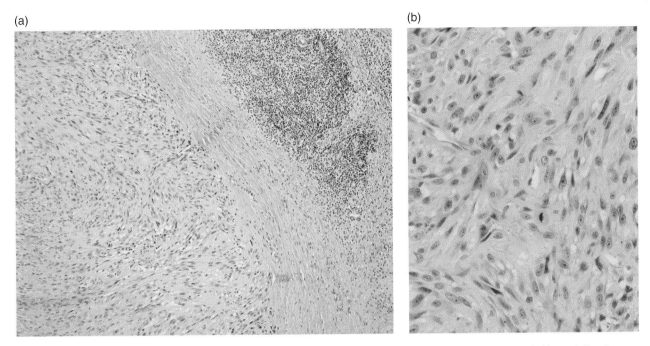

Figure 3.98   (a, b) Feline vaccination site sarcoma. This is an aggressive fibrosarcoma that is typically surrounded by multifocal aggregates of lymphocytes.

Cutaneous Hemangiosarcoma   This is a malignant invasive mass in the dermis that is composed of spindle cells, some of which are forming spaces filled with blood. The neoplastic cells have an oval nucleus, 1–2 nucleoli, a moderate amount of eosinophilic cytoplasm, and an indistinct cell border. There is moderate anisocytosis and anisokaryosis with occasional bizarre cells and a high mitotic index (Figure 3.100a, b).

Round Cell Neoplasms and Reactive Proliferations

Cutaneous Lymphoma

Cutaneous lymphoma is a form of lymphoma that involves only or predominantly the skin and occurs most commonly in dogs and horses. It may have a variable gross appearance, from nodular masses in the dermis to plaque-like thickening of the epidermis, and can have either a B-cell or T-cell immunophenotype. Also, skin involvement may be a manifestation of multicentric lymphoma. **Epidermotropic lymphoma** occurs primarily in dogs; it is a multifocal lesion that may also involve the epithelium of the adnexa and lips. It is a form of T-cell lymphoma in which the epidermis is thickened and contains a marked multifocal infiltrate of large round cells that sometimes form aggregates. These cells have a single oval to reniform nucleus, a prominent nucleolus, a moderate rim of pale eosinophilic or clear cytoplasm, and distinct cell borders. Neoplastic cells are also frequently present in the epithelium of the hair follicles and apocrine glands and may extend into the superficial dermis. The mitotic rate is moderate to high (Figure 3.101a, b).

Cutaneous Histiocytic Diseases

This is a group of cutaneous diseases that are characterized by reactive (non-neoplastic) or neoplastic proliferation of dendritic cells, either Langerhans (intraepidermal) dendritic cells or interstitial/perivascular dendritic cells. Several of these conditions may extend to internal organs. These conditions are most common in dogs. However, there are two histiocytic diseases that may occur in the skin and subcutis of cats, **Feline Progressive Histiocytosis (FPH)** and **Feline Histiocytic Sarcoma (FHS)**; both of which are derived from interstitial dendritic cells.

Canine Cutaneous Histiocytoma   This is a benign neoplasm of Langerhans dendritic cells unique to dogs and most commonly occurs in dogs that are three years old or younger, although they may occur at any age. They are usually seen as a small domed, or button-shaped, circumscribed, solitary nodule. Microscopically, they are composed of an intradermal sheet of round cells with eccentric round to reniform nuclei admixed with numerous aggregates of lymphocytes and plasma cells,

(a)

(b)

(c)

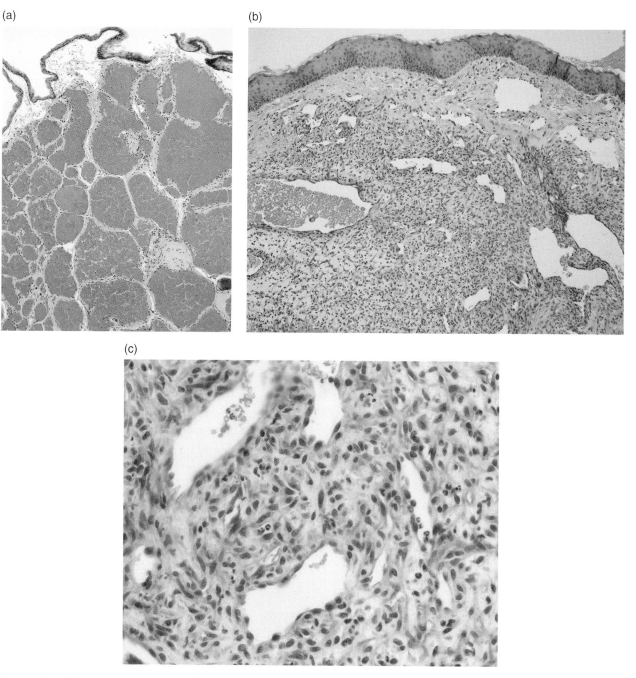

Figure 3.99 (a) Cavernous hemangioma. This is composed of multiple blood-filled vascular spaces lined by a single layer of flattened endothelium. (b, c) Granulation tissue type hemangioma. This pattern lacks substantial vascular spaces but instead is composed of spindle cells, some of which are forming small indistinct spaces filled with blood.

especially along the deep margin. The mitotic index is high, but there is minimal anisocytosis and anisokaryosis. In addition, there are frequently foci of necrosis scattered throughout the mass, especially those neoplasms that are in the process of regressing. The surface is often ulcerated and covered with a serocellular crust (Figure 3.102a–c).

Canine Persistent and Recurrent Cutaneous Histiocytomas

This is an uncommon form of histiocytoma that has multiple cutaneous nodules; a few may regress, but many do not. These nodules are also composed of Langerhans dendritic cells and microscopically resemble a typical histiocytoma, although they contain more plasma cells and few T-lymphocytes. Occasionally, this proliferative cell population will extend

(a)

(b)

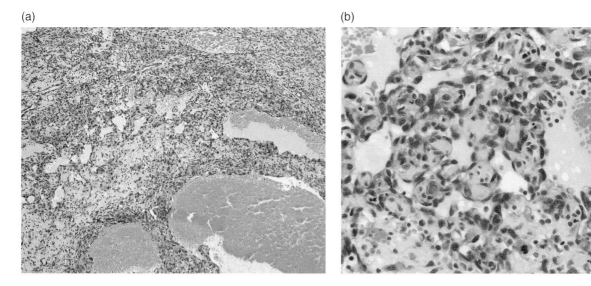

Figure 3.100   (a, b) Cutaneous hemangiosarcoma.

(a)

(b)

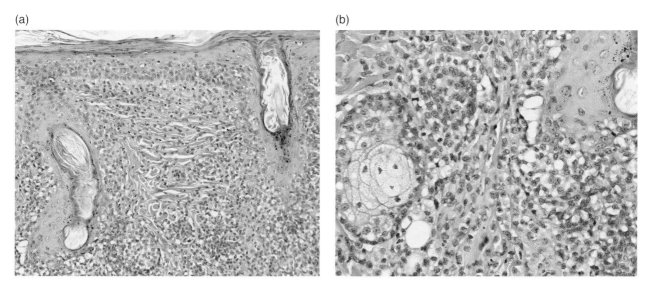

Figure 3.101   (a, b) Epidermotropic lymphoma. Neoplastic T-cells invade the epidermis and adnexa.

into draining lymph nodes and other internal organs; when this occurs, the condition is termed **Langerhans Cell Histiocytosis** and has a poor prognosis.

Canine Cutaneous and Systemic Reactive Histiocytosis   This is a rare proliferative histiocytic disorder that best fits the criteria of an idiopathic non-neoplastic condition. It is due to reactive proliferation of interstitial dendritic cells. There are two forms of this condition; one is cutaneous reactive histiocytosis and the other is systemic reactive histiocytosis. In the cutaneous form, there are typically multiple cutaneous nodules that tend to wax and wane; the systemic form has lesions in organs in addition to the skin. Bernese Mountain Dogs, Labrador retrievers and Golden retrievers are several breeds with an apparent predisposition for the systemic form. Microscopically, there are nodules in the deep dermis and panniculus that are composed of sheets of round cells with an oval to reniform peripheral nucleus, abundant eosinophilic cytoplasm and discernible cell borders. In addition, there is a scattered infiltrate of lymphocytes and a few plasma cells. These sheets of round cells form linear aggregates that track along the adnexae to the panniculus. These aggregates coalesce along the

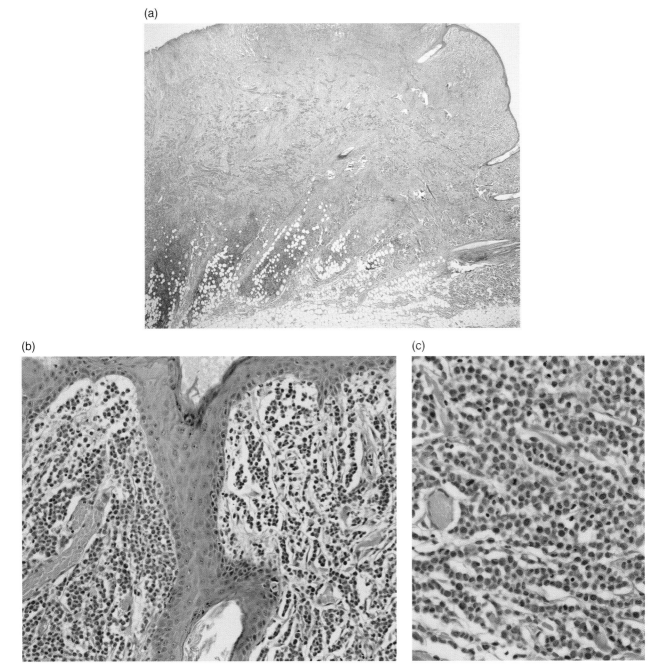

Figure 3.102 (a) Canine cutaneous histiocytoma. There is a dome-shaped accumulation of neoplastic round cells within the dermis. Also, there are commonly foci of necrosis throughout with an accumulation of lymphocytes along the deep margin. (b, c) Canine cutaneous histiocytoma. Neoplastic round cells are typically aligned in rows. These cells have a round to reniform nucleus and a moderate amount of eosinophilic cytoplasm.

deep margin within the panniculus, where they closely invest arterioles; there is limited angioinvasion in some of these deep areas. Also, there are a few scattered foci of necrosis within the deep areas. The mitotic index is high, and both forms are slowly progressive (Figure 3.103a, b).

Canine Histiocytic Sarcoma This may occur as a single neoplasm in one of several locations, including the skin and periarticular connective tissue, or as several neoplasms disseminated throughout the body, especially the liver, spleen, lymph nodes, and/or lung. The neoplastic cells are typically derived from interstitial dendritic cells, but there is also a

(a)
(b)

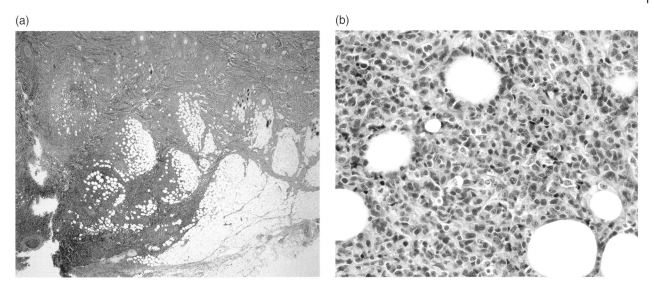

Figure 3.103   (a, b) Canine cutaneous and systemic reactive histiocytosis. There is a nodular accumulation of neoplastic round cells that somewhat track along the adnexa within the deep dermis, extending into the panniculus.

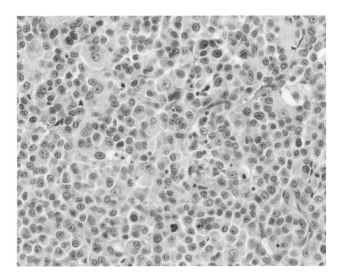

Figure 3.104   Canine histiocytic sarcoma. This is a poorly circumscribed mass in the dermis composed of a loose sheet of individualized round cells, which have an eccentric round to reniform nucleus, 1–2 nucleoli, a substantial amount of eosinophilic cytoplasm, and a distinct cell border. There is moderate to marked anisocytosis and anisokaryosis.

hemophagocytic form of HS in which the neoplastic cells are derived from bone marrow macrophages. Although HS can occur in any breed of dog, several breeds, most notably Bernese Mountain Dogs, Golden Retrievers, Flat-coated Retrievers and Rottweilers, are prone to develop HS. Microscopically, the cutaneous lesion is a poorly circumscribed mass in the dermis that is composed of a loose sheet of individualized round cells, which have an eccentric round to reniform nucleus, 1–2 nucleoli, a substantial amount of eosinophilic cytoplasm, and a distinct cell border. There is moderate to marked anisocytosis and anisokaryosis, frequently with multinucleate giant cells and a high mitotic index (Figure 3.104). Complete surgical clearance of the localized form of HS may be curative, but the disseminated form of HS has a poor prognosis.

Feline Progressive Histiocytosis   This initially forms one or more nodules in the dermis and panniculus, which are composed of well-differentiated, round to oval cells with a central oval to reniform nucleus, a nucleolus, a moderate to substantial amount of eosinophilic cytoplasm, and a distinct cell border. There is minimal to moderate anisocytosis and anisokaryosis with occasional multinucleate cells and a moderate to high mitotic index. Occasionally, histiocytic cells may be in the

(a)

(b)

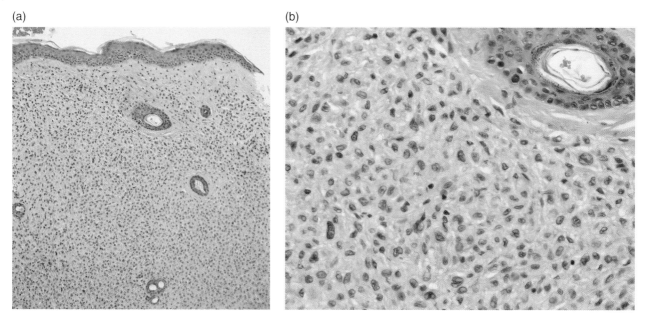

Figure 3.105 (a, b) Feline progressive histiocytosis. This forms nodules in the dermis that are composed of well-differentiated, round to oval cells with a central oval to reniform nucleus, a nucleolus, a moderate to substantial amount of eosinophilic cytoplasm, and a distinct cell border. There is minimal to moderate anisocytosis and anisokaryosis with occasional multinucleate cells and a moderate to high mitotic index.

epidermis. Over time, the histiocytic cells in these nodules progressively become more pleomorphic; these may also spread to lymph nodes and other internal organs, resembling histiocytic sarcoma (Figure 3.105a, b).

Feline Histiocytic Sarcoma   This may involve the skin or periarticular connective tissue, as well as internal organs. It is similar to HS in dogs, although less common. The lesions are invasive, poorly-circumscribed masses composed of a sheet of individualized round to polyhedral to spindle cells, which have a round to reniform nucleus, 1–2 nucleoli, a substantial amount of eosinophilic cytoplasm, and a distinct cell border. Many cells have multiple nuclei, and there is typically marked anisocytosis and anisokaryosis. The mitotic index is high with bizarre mitotic figures. In addition, there may be a modest infiltrate of lymphocytes and plasma cells (Figure 3.106a, b). The long-term prognosis is guarded to poor due to the progressive nature of the disease.

Cutaneous Plasmacytoma

Cutaneous Plasmacytoma is a neoplasm of plasma cell lineage that is typically located in the dermis, including the pinna, external ear canal, and digits. Cutaneous plasmacytomas are usually benign; however, some variants have been reported to metastasize to regional nodes. These are usually a circumscribed, nonencapsulated mass that is composed of round to pyriform cells with an eccentric round to reniform nucleus, a moderate amount of eosinophilic to basophilic cytoplasm, a distinct cell boundary and are aligned in sheets or small packets. There is moderate anisocytosis, anisokaryosis, numerous binucleate cells and cells with giant nuclei, and a moderate to high mitotic index (Figure 3.107a, b).

Canine Cutaneous Mast Cell Tumors

Canine cutaneous mast cell tumors are very common tumors. Certain breeds of dogs, such as Boston Terriers and Boxers, have a predilection for developing cutaneous mast cell tumors. Potential for metastasis varies with the degree of differentiation of the neoplastic cells: the better the degree of differentiation, the less likely they are to metastasize. The most current grading system (2 tier system) categorizes cutaneous mast cell tumors as either low-grade or high-grade based on the degree of differentiation, cellular pleomorphism, and mitotic index. **Low-grade mast cell tumors** are somewhat circumscribed, nonencapsulated masses in the dermis that may extend into the panniculus. They are typically composed of individualized round cells aligned in sheets and cords. These cells have a round to reniform central nucleus, a small nucleolus, a substantial amount of finely granular basophilic cytoplasm and a somewhat ragged cell border. In addition, there is

(a)

(b)

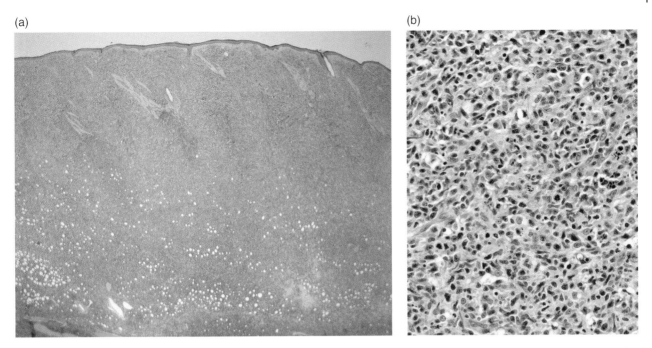

Figure 3.106 (a, b) Feline histiocytic sarcoma. This is an invasive, poorly-circumscribed mass composed of a sheet of individualized round to polyhedral to spindle cells, which have a round to reniform nucleus, 1–2 nucleoli, a substantial amount of eosinophilic cytoplasm and a distinct cell border. Many cells have multiple nuclei, and there is typically marked anisocytosis and anisokaryosis.

(a)

(b)

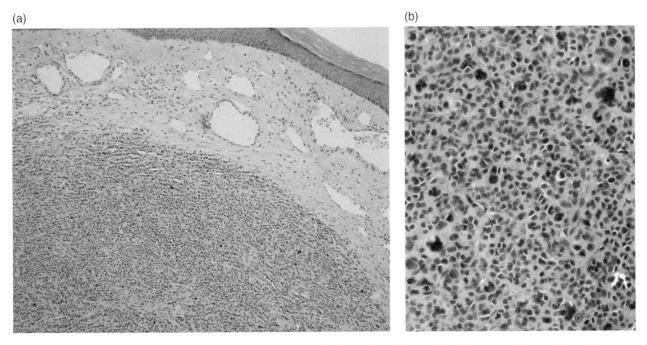

Figure 3.107 (a, b) Cutaneous plasmacytoma. These are composed of round to pyriform cells with an eccentric round to reniform nucleus, a moderate amount of eosinophilic to basophilic cytoplasm, a distinct cell boundary and are aligned in sheets or small packets. There is moderate anisocytosis, anisokaryosis, numerous binucleate cells and cells with giant nuclei, and a moderate to high mitotic index.

(a)

(b)

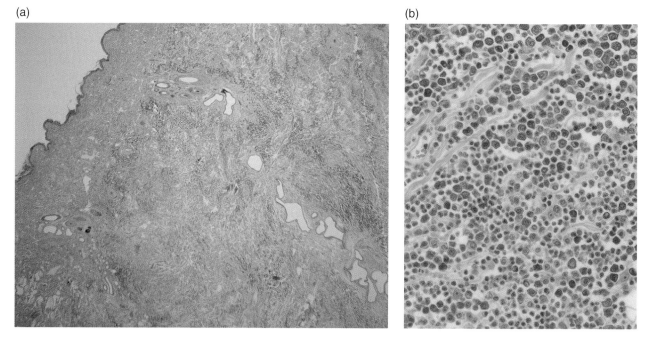

Figure 3.108   (a, b) Canine cutaneous mast cell tumor, low-grade. This is composed of a sheet of individualized, heavily-granulated mast cells with little anisocytosis and anisokaryosis, with a low mitotic index.

usually a diffuse infiltrate of eosinophils throughout. The mitotic index is low (<1/10 400× fields), and there is minimal anisocytosis and anisokaryosis (Figure 3.108a, b). In contrast, tumors are considered high-grade if they have at least one of the following characteristics: a mitotic index >7/10 400× fields; 3 multinucleate cells/10 400× fields; 3 bizarre nuclei/10 400X fields; or karyomegaly of 10% of the neoplastic cells. **High-grade mast cell tumors** are invasive, poorly- circumscribed, nonencapsulated masses in the dermis and frequently panniculus that are composed of individualized round cells, occasionally aligned in sheets or cords. These cells have a round to reniform central nucleus, 1–2 nucleoli, a substantial amount of basophilic cytoplasm that frequently contain a diminished number of metachromatic granules and a somewhat ragged cell border. The mitotic index is high (>7/10 400× fields), and there is moderate to marked anisocytosis and anisokaryosis with multinucleate cells and karyomegaly in some areas. There is also a variable infiltrate of eosinophils, some of which may be surrounding foci of hyalinized, fragmented collagen (Figure 3.109). Low-grade tumors have little potential for

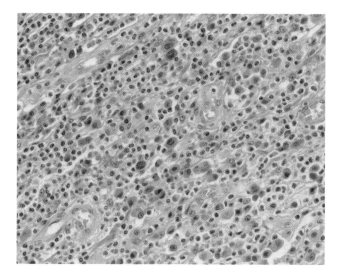

Figure 3.109   Canine cutaneous mast cell tumor, high-grade. This is composed of a pleomorphic population of variably-granulated mast cells, some of which are binucleate with a high mitotic index.

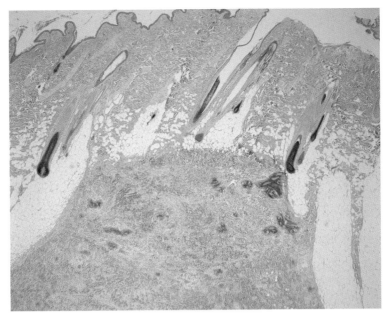

Figure 3.110 Canine subcutaneous mast cell tumor. This has features similar to cutaneous mast cell tumors but is primarily located in the panniculus. These may contain foci of hyalinized, fragmented collagen (flame figures) surrounded by eosinophils.

metastasis, and complete surgical clearance (margins of 2–5 mm) is curative; the median survival time is >two years. The median survival time for dogs with high-grade tumors is four months or less, and metastasis to regional lymph nodes is common; local recurrence is also common because determining surgical clearance with confidence can be difficult.

Canine Subcutaneous Mast Cell Tumors

Canine subcutaneous mast cell tumors are also common tumors but less common than cutaneous tumors. The 2 Tier grading system used for canine cutaneous mast cell tumors does not apply to subcutaneous tumors. Over 90% are benign, and complete surgical clearance is curative. Microscopically, these resemble low-grade cutaneous tumors except they originate in the adipose tissue of the panniculus (Figure 3.110).

Feline Cutaneous Mast Cell Tumors

Feline cutaneous mast cell tumors are typically benign neoplasms. They may be single or multiple and are most common on the head and neck. Microscopically, there are three patterns recognized: well-differentiated, pleomorphic, and atypical (also called histiocytic). Most cutaneous feline mast tumors are the well-differentiated pattern and are circumscribed, nonencapsulated masses in the dermis and panniculus that are composed of a sheet of round to polygonal cells that have a round to oval central nucleus, 1–2 small nucleoli, abundant finely granular eosinophilic cytoplasm, and distinct cell borders. There is minimal anisocytosis and a low mitotic index (<1/10 400× fields). They also frequently contain a few scattered eosinophils and aggregates of lymphocytes throughout the mass (Figure 3.111a, b). **Pleomorphic mast cell tumors** have moderate to marked anisocytosis and anisokaryosis with karyomegaly and a more substantial infiltrate of eosinophils (Figure 3.112). **Atypical (histiocytic) mast cell tumors** have a monomorphic population of individualized, moderately large round to polygonal cells with an oval to reniform nucleus and abundant eosinophilic cytoplasm with few granules (Figure 3.113a, b). A high mitotic index is not common in any of these patterns, but when present, it indicates more aggressive behavior.

Equine Cutaneous Mast Cell Tumors

Equine cutaneous mast cell tumors are uncommon benign neoplasms. Microscopically, they are circumscribed, nonencapsulated masses, composed of multiple sheets of round, somewhat individualized well-differentiated mast cells that have a round central nucleus, a prominent nucleolus, a substantial amount of basophilic granular cytoplasm, and distinct cell borders. In addition, these sheets of neoplastic cells contain a diffuse infiltrate of eosinophils and may be subdivided by bands of dense fibrous tissue. Also, these neoplasms frequently contain numerous large aggregates of degenerate eosinophils associated with foci of collagen fragmentation and necrosis (Figure 3.114a, b).

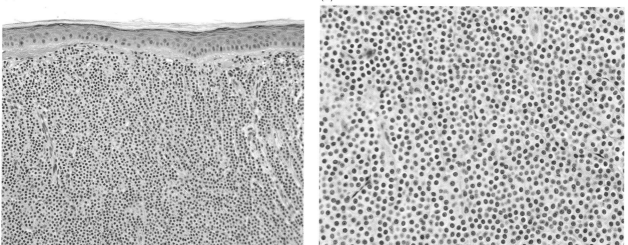

Figure 3.111 (a, b) Feline mast cell tumor. This is composed of a sheet of round to polygonal cells that have a round to oval central nucleus, 1–2 small nucleoli, abundant finely granular eosinophilic cytoplasm, and distinct cell borders. There is minimal anisocytosis, a low mitotic index. Also, there is typically a modest infiltrate of eosinophils and aggregates of lymphocytes.

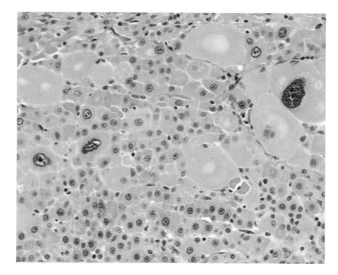

Figure 3.112 Feline pleomorphic mast cell tumor. This is composed of round to polygonal cells with moderate to marked anisocytosis and anisokaryosis with karyomegaly and a more substantial infiltrate of eosinophils.

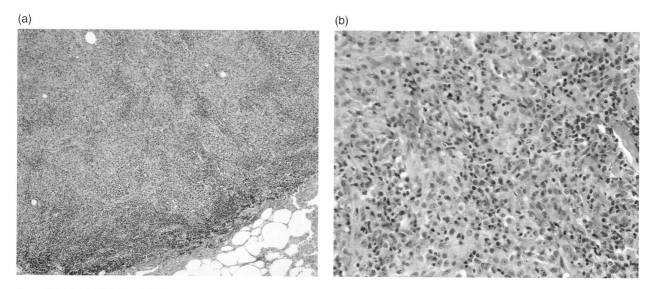

Figure 3.113 (a, b) Feline histiocytic mast cell tumor. This has a monomorphic population of individualized, moderately large round to polygonal cells with an oval to reniform nucleus and abundant eosinophilic cytoplasm with few granules.

(a)

(b)

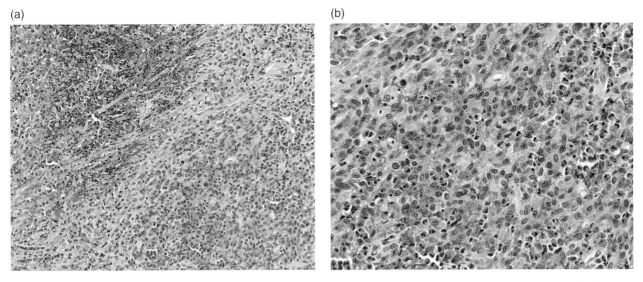

Figure 3.114 (a, b) Equine cutaneous mast cell tumor. This is composed of multiple sheets of round, somewhat individualized well-differentiated mast cells that have a round central nucleus, a prominent nucleolus, a substantial amount of basophilic granular cytoplasm, and distinct cell borders. In addition, there is an infiltrate of eosinophils, which are frequently associated with foci of necrosis with collagen hyalinization and fragmentation.

Other Masses, Cysts, and Cyst-like Structures

Follicular Cyst

Follicular cyst is the general term for a cystic dermal lesion that has the characteristics of a hair follicle. These are common benign lesions in dogs and less common in cats. They are composed of a lining of stratified squamous epithelium with characteristics of the epithelium that line the various levels or a hair follicle, the infundibulum, isthmus, and hair bulb, and have a lumen that is filled with keratinaceous debris. There are several subtypes of follicular cysts that are based on the characteristics of the lining epithelium. It is common for follicular cysts to be bordered by granulomatous or pyogranulomatous inflammation in response leakage of lumen contents following partial cyst rupture.

Infundibular Cyst
This is lined by stratified squamous epithelium that has a granular layer (Figure 3.115).

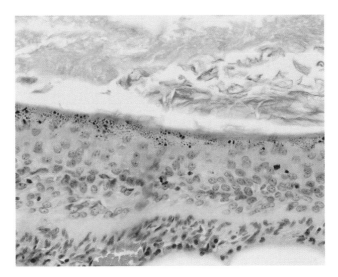

Figure 3.115 Infundibular follicular cyst. This type of cyst is lined by stratified squamous epithelium that has a granular layer.

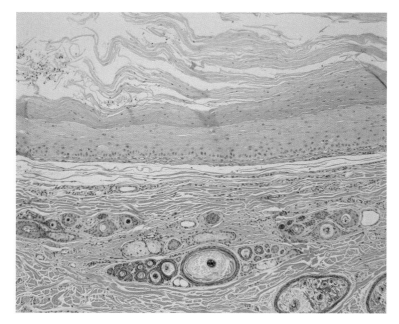

Figure 3.116   Isthmus follicular cyst. This type of cyst is lined by stratified squamous epithelium that lacks a granular layer.

Isthmus Cyst

This is lined by stratified squamous epithelium that lacks a granular layer (Figure 3.116).

Matrical Cyst

This is a multilocular cyst lined by a proliferative layer of basal cells that have abrupt transition into rafts of ghost cells (i.e. necrotic squamous epithelial cells). This is considered to be a cystic variant of a pilomatricoma (Figure 3.117).

Hybrid Cyst

This is a cyst that is lined by a combination of stratified squamous and basal epithelium. In some areas, there may be a stratum granulosum, but in other areas there is not. The lumen is filled with keratinaceous debris along with necrotic keratinized epithelium, some of which forms sheets of ghost cells, which may be pigmented (Figure 3.118a, b).

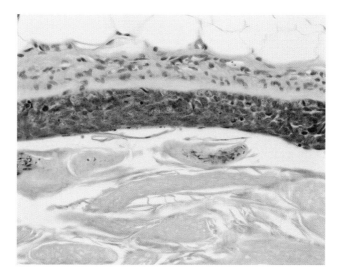

Figure 3.117   Matrical cyst. This is lined by a proliferative layer of basal cells that have abrupt transition into rafts of ghost cells (i.e. necrotic squamous epithelial cells).

(a)

(b)

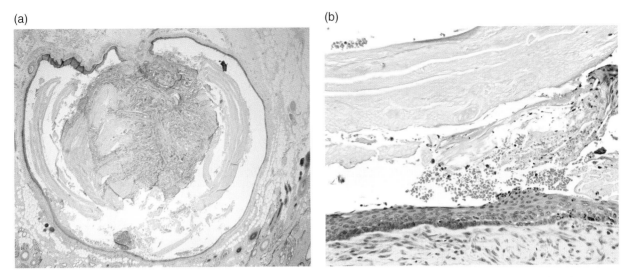

Figure 3.118   (a, b) Hybrid cyst. This is a cyst that is lined by a combination of stratified squamous and basal epithelium. In some areas, there may be a stratum granulosum, but in other areas, there is not. The lumen is filled with keratinaceous debris along with necrotic keratinized epithelium some of which forms sheets of ghost cells.

Dermoid Cyst

Dermoid cyst is a cystic cutaneous lesion that is lined by intact epidermis along with pilosebaceous units and is surrounded by a layer of dense irregular collagen. The lumen is filled with keratinaceous debris and hair. There is frequently a communication to the skin surface via a pore (Figure 3.119a, b). These are benign lesions that are considered to be developmental anomalies associated with cutaneous closure defects, and therefore are typically in young dogs located along the dorsal midline.

Apocrine Gland Cyst

Apocrine gland cyst is a single or multilocular non-neoplastic lesion derived from cystic dilation of an apocrine gland. The cyst is lined by a single layer of cuboidal epithelium and has a lumen that is filled with pale secretion, which is frequently washed out during tissue processing. The lining epithelium may have decapitation buds on the luminal surface or may be somewhat attenuated due to compression from the luminal contents (Figure 3.120a, b).

(a)

(b)

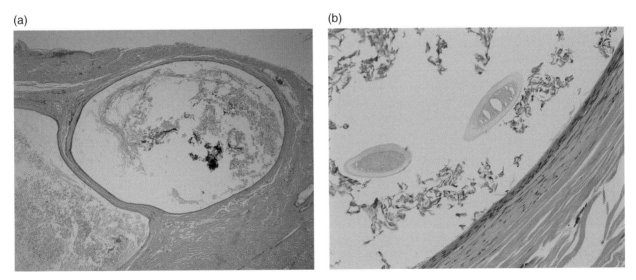

Figure 3.119   (a, b) Dermoid cyst. This is a cutaneous cystic lesion that is lined by intact epidermis along with pilosebaceous units and is surrounded by a layer of dense irregular collagen. The lumen is filled with keratinaceous debris and hair.

(a) (b)

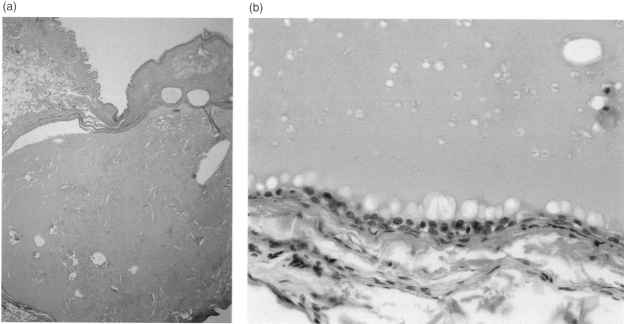

Figure 3.120   (a, b) Apocrine cyst. This is a dilated apocrine gland that is lined by a layer of apocrine epithelium and filled with eosinophilic secretion.

Canine Apocrine Cystomatosis

Canine apocrine cystomatosis is an idiopathic, non-neoplastic condition characterized by multiple apocrine cysts aligned in clusters within the skin. Microscopically, the cysts are similar to single apocrine cysts.

Feline Ceruminous Cystomatosis

Feline ceruminous cystomatosis is an idiopathic, non-neoplastic condition characterized by multiple cystic ceruminous glands aligned in clusters within the skin of the external ear canal and inner surface of the pinna. The cystic glands are lined by a single layer of cuboidal to columnar epithelium, and their lumens are filled with reddish-brown secretion, characteristic of ceruminous glands (Figure 3.121).

Calcinosis Circumscripta

Calcinosis circumscripta is a common idiopathic multilocular cutaneous lesion that occurs in dogs and is composed of numerous aggregates of mineralized material surrounded by a layer of macrophages and multinucleate giant cells. These aggregates are separated by fibrous tissue (Figure 3.122a, b). It is a form of tumoral calcinosis and is found most commonly on the limbs, especially at the elbow; it also occurs in the tongue.

Follicular Hamartoma

Follicular hamartoma is a non-neoplastic focal accumulation of large, normally-oriented anagen hair follicles and associated adnexae.

Fibroadnexal Hamartoma

Fibroadnexal hamartoma is a common non-neoplastic proliferation of fibrous tissue around displaced and disorganized hair follicles and adnexae. The hair follicles are typically dilated and lack hair bulbs (Figure 3.123). This may be a developmental anomaly or more likely, the result of a previous cutaneous injury.

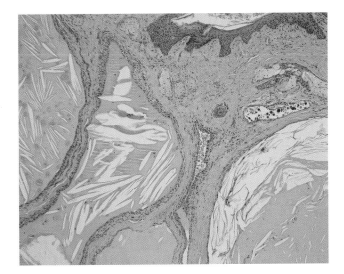

Figure 3.121 Feline ceruminous cystomatosis. This is characterized by multiple cystic ceruminous glands aligned in clusters within the skin of the external ear canal and inner surface of the pinna. The cystic glands are lined by a single layer of cuboidal to columnar epithelium, and their lumens are filled with reddish-brown secretion, characteristic of ceruminous glands.

(a)

(b)

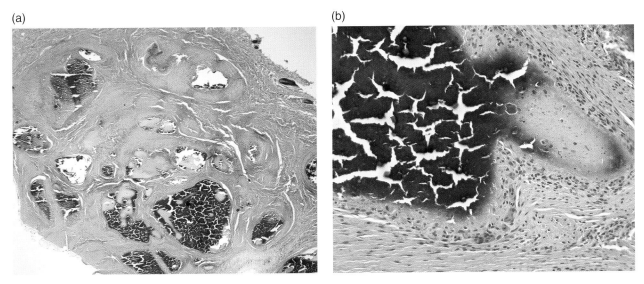

Figure 3.122 (a, b) Calcinosis circumscripta. This cutaneous lesion is composed of numerous aggregates of mineralized material surrounded by a layer of macrophages and multinucleate giant cells.

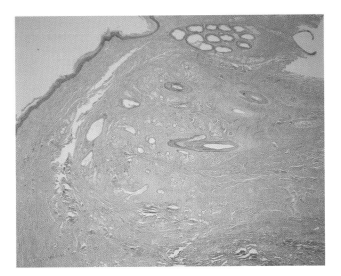

Figure 3.123 Fibroadnexal hamartoma. This is a proliferation of fibrous tissue around displaced and disorganized hair follicles and adnexae. The hair follicles may be dilated and lack hair bulbs.

Collagenous Hamartoma

Collagenous hamartoma is a poorly-circumscribed, non-neoplastic mass of dense irregular fibrous tissue with low cellularity in the dermis associated with a few displaced, dilated hair follicles (Figure 3.124).

Acrochordon (Skin Tag)

Acrochordon (skin tag) is a non-neoplastic polypoid mass that protrudes from the skin and is composed of a core of dense irregular fibrous tissue and a covering of moderately hyperplastic epidermis (Figure 3.125). These generally lack adnexal structures.

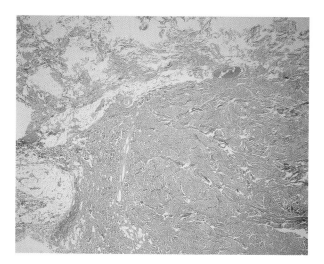

Figure 3.124 Collagenous hamartoma. This is a poorly-circumscribed, non-neoplastic mass of dense irregular fibrous tissue with low cellularity in the dermis.

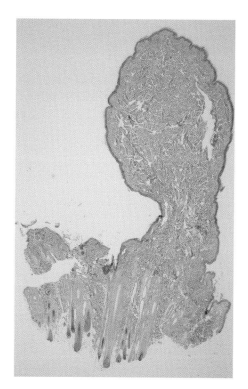

Figure 3.125 Acrochordon (skin tag). This is a non-neoplastic polypoid mass that protrudes from the skin and is composed of a core of dense irregular fibrous tissue and a covering of moderately hyperplastic epidermis.

References and Additional Readings

Bellamy, E. and Berlato, D. (2021). Canine cutaneous and subcutaneous mast cell tumours: a review. *J. Small Anim. Pract.* https://doi.org/10.1111/jsap.13444.

Bryden, S.L., White, S.D., Dunston, S.M. et al. (2005 Aug). Clinical, histopathological and immunological characteristics of exfoliative cutaneous lupus erythematosus in 25 German short-haired pointers. *Vet. Dermatol.* 16 (4): 239–252. https://doi.org/10.1111/j.1365-3164.2005.00468.x.

Coste, M., Prata, D., Castiglioni, V. et al. (2019). Feline progressive histiocytosis: a retrospective investigation of 26 cases and preliminary study of Ki67 as a prognostic marker. *J. Vet. Diagn. Invest.* 31 (6): 801–808. https://doi.org/10.1177/1040638719884950.

Gross, T.L., Halliwell, R.E., McDougal, B.J., and Rosencrantz, W.S. (1986 Jan). Psoriasiform lichenoid dermatitis in the springer spaniel. *Vet. Pathol.* 23 (1): 76–78. https://doi.org/10.1177/030098588602300113.

Gross, T.L., Song, M.D., Havel, P.J., and Ihrke, P.J. (1993 Jan). Superficial necrolytic dermatitis (necrolytic migratory erythema) in dogs. *Vet. Pathol.* 30 (1): 75–81. https://doi.org/10.1177/030098589303000110.

Hendrick, M.J. and Dunagan, C.A. (1991). Focal necrotizing granulomatous panniculitis associated with subcutaneous injection of rabies vaccine in cats and dogs: 10 cases (1988–1989). *J. Am. Vet. Med. Assoc.* 198 (2): 304–305.

Maxie, M.G. (ed.) (2016). Chapter 6 – Integumentary system: Elizabeth Mauldin and Jeanine Peters-Kennedy. In: *Jubb, Kennedy and Palmer's pathology of domestic animals*, 6e, vol. 1, 509–736.

Kim, J.H., Kang, K.I., Sohn, H.J. et al. (2005 Sep). Color-dilution alopecia in dogs. *J. Vet. Sci.* 6 (3): 259–261. PMID: 16131833.

Kiupel, M. and Camus, M. (2019 Sep). Diagnosis and prognosis of canine cutaneous mast cell Tumors. *Vet. Clin. North Am. Small Anim. Pract.* 49 (5): 819–836. https://doi.org/10.1016/j.cvsm.2019.04.002.

Mikaelian, I. and Gross, T.L. (2002 Jan). Keloidal fibromas and fibrosarcomas in the dog. *Vet. Pathol.* 39 (1): 149–153. https://doi.org/10.1354/vp.39-1-149.

Miller, M.A. and Dunstan, R.W. (1993). Seasonal flank alopecia in boxers and Airedale terriers: 24 cases (1985–1992). *J. Am. Vet. Med. Assoc.* 203 (11): 1567–1572. PMID: 8288480.

Moore, P.F. (2014 Jan). A review of histiocytic diseases of dogs and cats. *Vet. Pathol.* 51 (1): 167–184. https://doi.org/10.1177/0300985813510413.

Nishifuji, K., Park, S.J., and Iwasaki, T. (2007). A case of hyperplastic dermatosis of the West Highland White terrier controlled by recombinant canine interferon-gamma therapy. *J. Vet. Med. Sci.* 69 (4): 455–457. https://doi.org/10.1292/jvms.69.455.

Olivry, T. (2006). A review of autoimmune skin diseases in domestic animals: I – superficial pemphigus. *Vet. Dermatol.* 17 (5): 291–305. https://doi.org/10.1111/j.1365-3164.2006.00540.x.

Porcellato, I., Menchetti, L., Brachelente, C. et al. (2017). Feline injection-site sarcoma. *Vet. Pathol.* 54 (2): 204–211. https://doi.org/10.1177/0300985816677148.

Psalla, D., Rüfenacht, S., Stoffel, M.H. et al. (2013 Nov). Equine pastern vasculitis: a clinical and histopathological study. *Vet. J.* 198 (2): 524–530. https://doi.org/10.1016/j.tvjl.2013.09.001.

Simpson, A. and McKay, L. (2012 Oct). Applied dermatology: sebaceous adenitis in dogs. *Compend. Contin. Educ. Vet.* 34 (10): E1–E7. PMID: 23532758.

Goldschmidt, M. and Goldschmidt, K. (2017). Chapter 4 – Epithelial and melanocytic tumors of skin. In: *Tumors in Domestic Animals*, 5e (ed. D. Meuten), 88–141.

Hendrick, M. (2017). Chapter 5 – Mesenchymal tumors of the skin and soft tissues. In: *Tumors in Domestic Animals*, 142–175.

Kiupel, M. (2017). Chapter 6 – Mast Cell Tumors. In: *Tumors in Domestic Animals*, 176–202.

White, S.D., Bourdeau, P., Rosychuk, R.A. et al. (2001 Apr). Zinc-responsive dermatosis in dogs: 41 cases and literature review. *Vet. Dermatol.* 12 (2): 101–109. https://doi.org/10.1046/j.1365-3164.2001.00233.x.

Yager, J.A. (2014). Erythema multiforme, Stevens-Johnson syndrome and toxic epidermal necrolysis: a comparative review. *Vet. Dermatol.* 25 (5): 406–e64. https://doi.org/10.1111/vde.12142.

4

Pathology of the Male Reproductive System

Michael J. Yaeger

Department of Veterinary Pathology, Iowa State University, Ames, IA, USA

Prostate

Introduction

There is considerable anatomic, chemical, and physiologic diversity of the prostate gland among mammalian species. The glands major role is the production of prostatic fluid, which has antibacterial properties and aids in supporting and transporting sperm during ejaculation. The only veterinary species that develop prostatic disorders with any frequency is the dog, where the disease is relatively common in older, intact, large-breed males.

The prostate is a compound tubular to the tubuloalveolar exocrine gland. The secretory alveoli are lined by simple columnar epithelial cells that have basally located nuclei and abundant eosinophilic cytoplasm with prominent apical cytoplasmic granules. In the dog, the alveolar portions of the gland contain primary and secondary infoldings of secretory epithelium, which project into the alveolar lumina. The alveoli are separated by a dense stroma that contains smooth muscle cells.

Developmental and Degenerative Diseases

Prostatic Hypoplasia/Atrophy
Castration of dogs at a young age removes the trophic endocrine factors necessary for prostatic development resulting in prostatic hypoplasia. Similarly, castration after the gland has fully developed leads to prostatic atrophy. Prostatic involution begins within days of castration and will be complete in 6–12 weeks. Neither hypoplasia nor atrophy is clinically relevant except as a method of disease prevention. Prostatic atrophy results in a smaller cross-sectional area of the gland, secretory epithelial cells will be decreased in height, their cytoplasmic content reduced, and the connective tissue stroma will become more prominent. Eventually, alveoli will be lined by flattened epithelial cells with small lumens (Figure 4.1).

Prostatic Hyperplasia/Hypertrophy
Prostatic hyperplasia is a spontaneous disease of intact male dogs that begins as early as three years of age. More than 50% of intact dogs will have evidence of prostatic hyperplasia by five years of age, 80% by the age of 6, and >95% by nine years of age. However, most intact males will not develop clinical signs associated with prostatic hyperplasia. When enlargement of the prostate gland causes clinical signs, fecal obstruction is typically observed, rather than urinary obstruction, as occurs in humans.

There are considered to be two histologic patterns of prostatic hyperplasia. These include glandular hyperplasia, which typically occurs in dogs under four years of age, and complex hyperplasia, which is identified in older dogs. Glandular hyperplasia is the result of epithelial hypertrophy and hyperplasia. There is an obvious increase in the amount of secretory epithelium. Each of the lobules will be larger and have more elaborate branching. In addition, the size of the secretory epithelial cells increases, principally due to an increase in the amount of cytoplasm.

Atlas of Veterinary Surgical Pathology, First Edition. Edited by Joseph S. Haynes.
© 2023 John Wiley & Sons, Inc. Published 2023 by John Wiley & Sons, Inc.

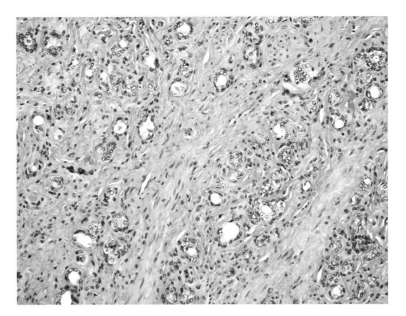

Figure 4.1   Prostatic atrophy. The secretory epithelial cells are decreased in height, their cytoplasmic content is reduced, the glandular lumen is diminished, and the connective tissue stroma, including smooth muscle, is more prominent.

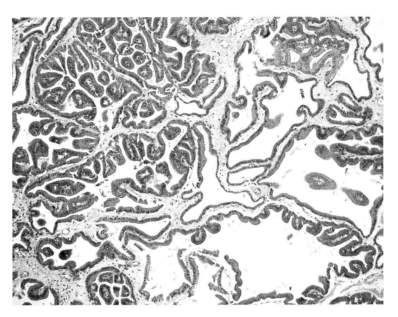

Figure 4.2   Prostatic hyperplasia. There is an increased amount of secretory epithelium with elaborate branching and papillary projections, cystic glandular dilation, and a mild increase in stromal fibrosis.

Complex hyperplasia is a combination of epithelial hyperplasia, cystic glandular dilation and mild stromal fibrosis. In complex hyperplasia, there is an increase in the relative lumen size of the glandular acini, typically accompanied by an increase in the volume of interstitial tissue, which is often mildly inflamed. There are often foci in which the secretory epithelium is atrophic and attenuated, accompanied by a relative increase in stroma comprising both collagen and smooth muscle. Some of the alveoli will be dilated and filled with eosinophilic material. These cysts are most often found in the periurethral area, although they can be present anywhere in the gland. The interstitium is often infiltrated by lymphocytes and plasma cells (Figure 4.2).

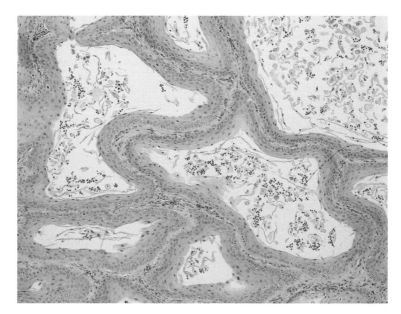

Figure 4.3   Squamous metaplasia of the prostate. Prostatic glands are lined by keratinizing stratified squamous epithelium. Glandular lumens contain sloughed squames, fine laminations of keratin, and scattered neutrophils.

Prostatic Cysts

The prevalence of prostatic cysts in adult large-breed dogs has been reported to be approximately 14%; of those, there was evidence of bacterial infection in 42% of the cases. Cysts may be congenital or secondary to any condition in which canaliculi become obstructed, leading to the accumulation of prostatic fluid, such as hyperplasia, neoplasia, or inflammation. Retention cysts are acquired cysts due to obstruction of the glandular ductules, causing retention of prostatic secretions and dilatation of affected acini. They are lined by flattened prostatic glandular epithelium or urothelium.

Prostatic Squamous Metaplasia

Squamous metaplasia of the prostatic epithelium is associated with elevated estrogenic activity, either as a result of exogenous administration or in association with estrogen secreting testicular tumors. Epithelial metaplasia involves the acini in all parts of the gland, the prostatic urethra, uterus masculinus, and ducts. The metaplastic stratified squamous epithelium exhibits progressive differentiation, and glandular lumens may contain sloughed squames or laminations of keratin. Glandular lumens also often contain macrophages and neutrophils. Epithelial squamous metaplasia is accompanied by an increase of the fibromuscular stroma. Squamous metaplasia may also occur secondary to prostatitis, but this change will be subtle, generally lacks keratinization, and will be associated with marked luminal inflammation (Figure 4.3).

Prostatic Inflammatory Diseases

Acute and Chronic Bacterial Prostatitis

Acute prostatitis typically affects mature male dogs. These animals often present with signs of systemic diseases, such as anorexia, fever, and depression, and may have a stiff or stilted gait, preputial discharge, and potentially an unwillingness to breed. Compromise of the prostate by hyperplasia, cysts, prostatic neoplasia, or squamous metaplasia may predispose to prostatic infection. The prostate may be colonized by bacteria that ascend up the urethra from the distal urinary tract, down the urethra from the urinary bladder, arrive from the infected epididymis or testes, or spread hematogenously. Systemic fungal infections, such as blastomycosis and cryptococcosis, are occasional causes of prostatitis in the dog. Acute prostatitis is typically characterized by infiltration of the interstitium, epithelium, and glandular lumens by neutrophils (Figure 4.4a, b).

Chronic prostatitis is more common than acute prostatitis, is more insidious in onset, and somewhat more difficult to detect, since many dogs present with vague clinical signs or lack clinical signs altogether. The most common presentation of dogs with chronic prostatitis is recurrent urinary tract infections or urethral discharge. Chronic bacterial prostatitis is characterized by expansion of the interstitium by lymphoplasmacytic infiltrates accompanied by increased interstitial fibrosis (Figure 4.5).

(a) (b)

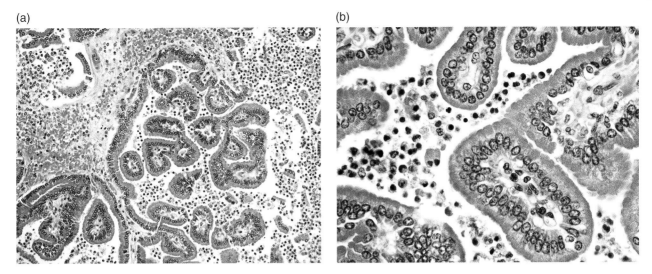

Figure 4.4   (a, b) Acute prostatitis. The glandular lumens are flooded by an exudate composed primarily of neutrophils. The glandular interstitium is moderately expanded by fibrin and hemorrhage.

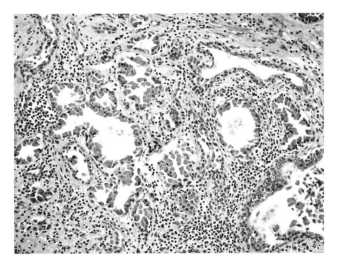

Figure 4.5   Chronic prostatitis. The glandular interstitium is moderately expanded by dense fibrous connective tissue infiltrated by moderate numbers of lymphocytes and lesser numbers of plasma cells.

Prostatic Abscessation

Prostatic abscesses may develop subsequent to suppurative prostatitis, secondary infection of prostatic cysts, or as a sequela to chronic prostatitis. Clinical signs may vary depending on the size of the abscess and whether the infection has become systemic. In dogs with very large prostatic abscesses, there may be signs of tenesmus or dysuria due to pressure on the colon or urethra, and a urethral discharge is common. Histologically, cavities of purulent fluid are found within the prostatic parenchyma.

Prostatic Neoplasia

The dog is the only species, other than man, that regularly develops spontaneous prostate cancer. Nonetheless, canine prostatic neoplasia is relatively rare, occurring in 5–7% of dogs with prostatic disease with an overall incidence of 0.2–0.6%. Prostatic neoplasia is the most commonly diagnosed prostatic disorder in castrated dogs. Neutered males have been reported to have an equal or greater risk of developing a prostatic tumor compared to intact dogs. Prostatic cancer in castrated dogs appears to have a more aggressive metastatic course.

Prostatic neoplasia is a disease of older dogs, with a mean age at diagnosis of 10 years. Common clinical signs include anorexia, weight loss, hematuria, stranguria, tenesmus, and potentially weakness in the rear limbs. On physical examination, affected individuals may have an asymmetric, firm, nodular, painful prostate. Metastasis to regional lymph nodes and pelvic bones is commonly associated with pain and neurological deficits in the pelvic limbs. The reported metastatic potential of these tumors is broad, ranging from 24 to 80% of cases at the time of diagnosis. These tumors have been reported to metastasize to a wide variety of tissues. One large study described lung (41.7%), regional lymph nodes (33.3%), and kidney (25%) as the most common metastatic sites, while another reported lymph node (64%), lung (62%), and bone (22%) as the most common sites for metastasis. Due to the difficulty in detecting skeletal metastasis, the true incidence of bone metastasis is likely higher. The lumbar vertebra, pelvis, and femur were the most frequently affected bones, with 95% of bone metastases located proximal to the elbow or knee.

Prostatic Adenocarcinoma

The most common tumors of the prostate are reported to be adenocarcinoma (51.8%), undifferentiated carcinoma (30.0%), and transitional cell carcinoma (TCC) (18.2%). Prostatic TCC, which arises from the prostatic urethra or prostatic ducts, is identified more commonly in castrated males. Squamous cell carcinoma (SCC), leiomyosarcoma, hemangiosarcoma, and lymphoma of the prostate have also been reported. Prostatic carcinoma has been classified into several types. Papillary: Tumors are composed of dilated ducts containing papillary projections of neoplastic cells with occasional central necrosis (comedonecrosis) (6% of tumors). Cribriform: Tumors are composed of ducts extended by neoplastic cells forming irregular fenestrae, often accompanied with central necrosis (16%). Solid (undifferentiated): Tumors are composed of solid sheets, cord of cells, or isolated individual cells lacking any specific histological growth pattern (16%). Small acinar/ductal: These tumors are composed of variably sized small acini and tubules admixed with moderate to the high amount of fibro-muscular stroma (24%). Signet ring: Neoplastic cells are arranged in sheets, small clusters, or as single cells and characterized by a clear cytoplasmic vacuole displacing the nucleus to one side. Signet ring cells must make up over 25% of the tumor volume. Mucinous: Adenocarcinoma with at least 25% of the tumor composed of lakes of extracellular mucin, with the exclusion of a nonprostatic origin; tumor growth patterns included cribriform, cords or strands, and tubules. For prostatic carcinomas, a single histologic pattern was identified in 62% of the tumors, whereas a mixture of histologic patterns was identified in 38% of prostatic carcinomas. Due to the heterogeneous histologic appearance of prostatic carcinomas in dogs and the current lack of a prostate-specific immunohistochemical marker suitable for canine tissues, it can be difficult to definitively differentiate canine prostatic TCCs from prostate carcinomas, leading to some authors recommending the use of the term carcinoma of the prostate (Figure 4.6a–c).

Prostatic Transitional Cell Carcinoma

Prostate TCC and prostatic carcinomas in dogs share morphologic features. Canine prostatic TCCs are composed of densely packed, moderately to markedly anaplastic epithelial cells arranged in solid, papillary, or cribriform patterns. The cells may form poorly arranged, highly cellular nests, acini, and tubules or cords, often in multiple layers. These tumors may be heterogeneous, with cell types ranging from small polyhedral cells with a high N:C ratio; a round, hyperchromatic nucleus; and scant eosinophilic cytoplasm to large cells with low N:C ratios; abundant eosinophilic cytoplasm; and round to ovoid, vesicular nuclei. Highly vacuolated and signet-ring cells are commonly seen in prostatic TCCs, and the vacuoles of these cells often contain a granular, basophilic material (Figure 4.7).

Testes and Epididymis

The primary functions of the testes are the production of hormones and sperm. Testicles are compound tubular glands surrounded by a thick, connective tissue capsule, the tunica albuginea, which has internal extensions that form fibrous partitions separating the testis into numerous lobules containing tightly-packed seminiferous tubules, which are the site of spermatogenesis. Seminiferous tubules are lined by two main cell types, Sertoli and spermatogenic cells. Sertoli cells form the blood–testis barrier and provide physical support for the developing sperm. In sexually mature animals, Sertoli cells make up only about 10% of the population lining seminiferous tubules, with germ cells comprise the bulk of the cells within the tubules. The testicular interstitium consists of loose connective tissue, blood and lymph vessels, free mononuclear cells, and polygonal interstitial endocrine (Leydig) cells that have eosinophilic cytoplasm containing small, clear lipid droplets.

(a)

(b)

(c)

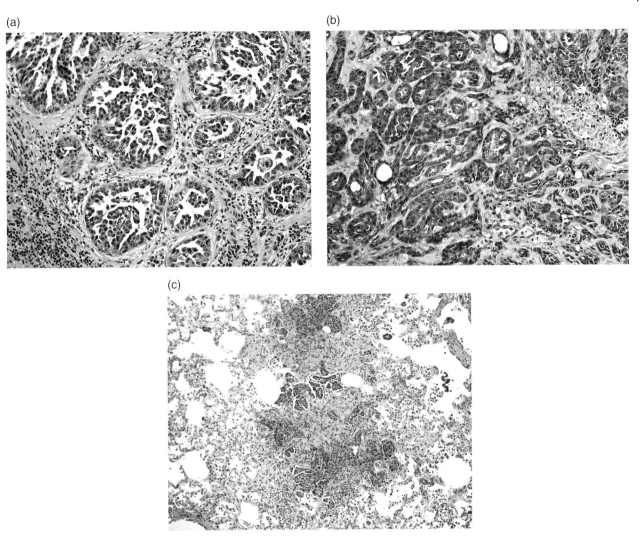

Figure 4.6 (a, b) Prostatic adenocarcinoma. The tumor is composed of a proliferation of epithelial cells arranged in irregular papillary projections (left) or a cribriform pattern (right). (c) Pulmonary metastasis of a prostatic adenocarcinoma

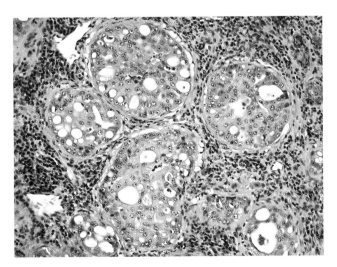

Figure 4.7 Prostatic transitional cell carcinoma. The tumor is composed of islands of epithelial cells variably arranged in solid clusters or surrounding small luminal spaces. Epithelial cells have abundant eosinophilic cytoplasm and round to ovoid, vesicular nuclei. There are occasional highly vacuolated and signet-ring cells. The adjacent interstitium is moderately expanded by an infiltrate of lymphocytes and plasma cells.

The epididymis is a single tube that is highly coiled where sperm is stored and matures. The ductal epithelium is pseudostratified columnar with stereocilia, and the interstitium contains layers of smooth muscle necessary to propel sperm along the ducts.

Testicular Hypoplasia

The hypoplastic testicle does not develop to its normal size and is always accompanied by epididymal hypoplasia. Cryptorchidism is the most commonly encountered disorder that leads to testicular and epididymal hypoplasia. In dogs, the incidence of cryptorchidism ranges between 0.8 and 15%, with pure bred dogs more commonly affected (77.5%). Unilateral cryptorchidism is more frequently detected in dogs (75%), and the right testis is involved twice more often. Feline cryptorchidism is uncommon having only been reported in 1.3–1.7% of male cats, and, similar to dogs, only one testicle is typically affected. Cryptorchidism is considered to be a sex-limited heritable trait transmitted by one or more autosomal genes. Cryptorchidism is common in male horses (2–8%), is most often unilateral (85–90%), occurs with equal frequency on either side and is generally accepted to be a hereditary condition. Maldescended testes exhibit varying degrees of hypoplasia and are predispose to neoplasia, spermatic cord torsion, and inguinal herniation.

The histological appearance of testicular hypoplasia is variable. In severely affected testes, all tubules lack germ cells or any evidence of spermatogenesis and are lined only by Sertoli cells. Other individuals have a lack of complete spermatogenesis with spermatogenesis stopping at a particular stage, such as at the primary spermatocyte stage. Hypoplastic testicles may have some normal tubules and some tubules that are arrested, often containing scattered apoptotic cells. Unfortunately, identical changes are observed in testicular degeneration, so other factors must be used to determine whether the changes are due to hypoplasia. Macroscopically, hypoplasia is distinguished from degeneration/atrophy because the epididymis in hypoplastic testes is proportionately small relative to the hypoplastic testis, whereas, in testicular atrophy, the epididymis is relatively large compared to the testis.

Testicular Atrophy/Degeneration

Testicular atrophy/degeneration may occur as a result of senescence, or following trauma, inflammation, toxin exposure, immune-mediated orchitis/epididymitis, overheating, neoplasia, infarction, obstruction, or an endocrinopathy. Age should always be considered when evaluating the testicle as hypoplastic/atrophic changes may also reflect immaturity in dogs less than eight months of age.

The main histological patterns reported for testicular degeneration/atrophy are seminiferous tubules that contain only Sertoli cells, completely lacking germ cells, and incomplete spermatogenesis with arrest of spermatogenesis at the stage of spermatogonia or of spermatocytes. In tubules with impaired spermatogenesis, Sertoli cells often have large empty intracytoplasmic vacuoles, which are lipid droplets and may be derived from phagocytosed germ cells. The majority of atrophic testes examined have histological evidence of some degree of impaired spermatogenesis, which is defined as "mixed atrophy." Multinucleated cells are often observed within the seminiferous tubules of atrophic canine testes. These cells arise from the fusion of germ cells or result from karyokinesis without cytokinesis and are considered an age-related finding. Immunohistochemical studies have shown re-expression of markers of immaturity in canine Sertoli cells and seminal cells in atrophic testes of dogs and men, suggesting that testicular atrophy may be a risk factor for tumor development (Figure 4.8a, b).

Infectious Orchitis and Epididymitis

Infectious orchitis/epididymitis can be caused by bacterial, fungal, or viral infection that may ascend from the urethra, descend from the prostate or bladder, arrive hematogenously, or enter via puncture wounds. Orchitis can be observed with feline infectious peritonitis in cats, *Corynebacterium pseudotuberculosis* in rams and bucks, and in stallions due to *Burkholderia pseudomallei*, salmonella septicemia, and migrating strongyle larvae. Canine epididymitis/orchitis is more common in young animals and may be caused by a wide variety of bacteria, viral, and fungal organisms, including *E. coli*, *Klebsiella* spp., *Pseudomonas* spp., *Staphylococcus* spp., *Streptococcus* spp., *Brucella* spp., *Mycoplasma* spp., *Ureaplasma* spp., paramyxoviruses, and *Blastomyces dermatitidis*.

(a)   (b)

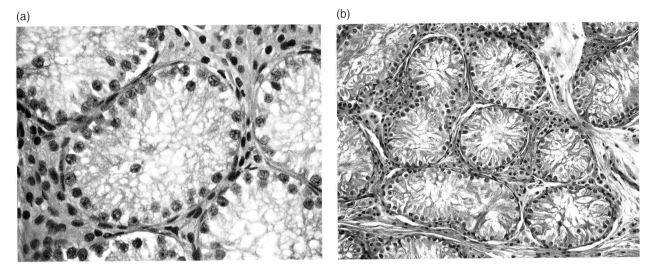

Figure 4.8   (a, b) Testicular atrophy and degeneration. The seminiferous tubules are lined primarily by Sertoli cells (left) or spermatogonia and Sertoli cells (right) and lack spermatogenesis.

Historically, orchitis/epididymitis in a variety of species has been linked with brucellosis and tuberculosis, which are no longer common but should not be disregarded. The most frequent manifestations of *Brucella* infection in the male reproductive tract are severe epididymitis and prostatitis, specifically lymphohistiocytic interstitial epididymitis, occasionally with evidence of intratubular neutrophils and spermatophagic macrophages; lymphohistiocytic funiculitis (spermatic cord); and lymphohistiocytic interstitial prostatitis. In dogs, testicular lesions are infrequent, variable, and may include chronic lymphohistiocytic orchitis with testicular fibrosis and atrophy, necrotizing vasculitis, and testicular necrosis. It is generally not possible to identify *Brucella* organisms with gram stains in the male reproductive tract.

Orchitis has been divided into three major categories: interstitial, intra-tubular, or necrotizing. Interstitial orchitis is characterized by the expansion of the intertubular stroma by fibrosis and lymphocytic inflammation. Intratubular orchitis most probably results from ascending infection and is characterized by retention of seminiferous tubule outlines, obliteration of lining cells, and intratubular accumulations of macrophages, neutrophils, and multinucleate giant cells. Necrotizing orchitis is typically the result of severe periorchitis reducing testicular blood flow leading to necrosis. Histologically, there will be extensive coagulation necrosis bordered by fibrosis and an intense inflammatory infiltrate. Regardless of the species or cause, chronic infection results in testicular and epididymal atrophy and fibrosis (Figure 4.9).

Spermatocele and Sperm Granulomas

A spermatocele is a cystic dilatation of the ductal system of the testis, epididymis, or vas deferens caused by loss of patency of a duct with stasis of sperm. Spermatoceles most commonly arise in the head of the epididymis and may be iatrogenic (vasectomy) or secondary to congenital anomalies, inflammation, or trauma. Rupture of the spermatocele with the release of spermatozoa leads to granulomatous inflammation (sperm granuloma). As a general rule, lesions in the caudal epididymis (tail) are more likely due to ascending infections, whereas granulomas in the head of the epididymis are more likely due to sperm granulomas.

The blood–testis barrier is one of the tightest blood–tissue barriers in the mammalian body isolating spermiogenesis from the body's immune system. Once the blood–testis barrier has been broken by trauma, infections, congenital abnormalities, degenerative changes, or toxins, the animal's immune system will recognize the body's sperm cells as foreign, leading to the development of spermatic granulomas. Spermatic granulomas consist of accumulations of spermatozoa and macrophages within tubules and/or in the adjacent interstitium (Figures 4.10a, b and 4.11).

Testicular Neoplasia

Dogs have the highest incidence of testicular tumors of all animal species. Testicular neoplasia tends to occur in aged male dogs (9–11 years) with a reported incidence of 0.91–5.8% in biopsy samples and 21–46% in necropsied, aged, male dogs. In 20–40% of testicles, multiple tumor types may be present in the same testicle, and tumors are bilateral in 28–38% of

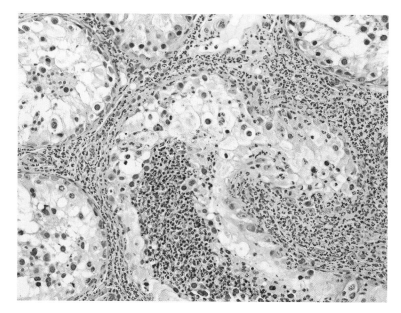

Figure 4.9 Suppurative orchitis. Seminiferous tubules contain a moderate suppurative exudate, there is a loss of the majority of lining cells, and a moderate infiltrate of neutrophils in the adjacent interstitium.

(a)

(b)

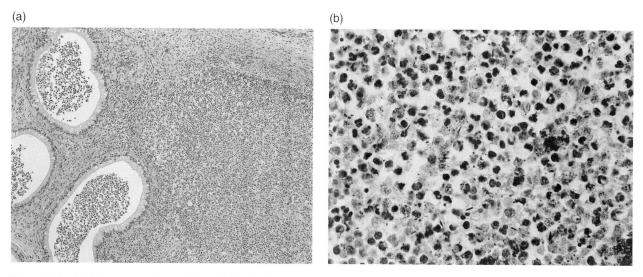

Figure 4.10 (a, b) Sperm granuloma. The epididymal ducts are moderately distended by a suppurative exudate. The interstitium is moderately expanded by connective tissue and infiltrated by neutrophils, macrophages, lymphocytes, and plasma cells. Focally, the interstitium is expanded by an intense infiltrate of neutrophils and macrophages (left). Basophilic linear degenerate spermatids (right) are present in the center of the pyogranuloma.

individuals. Similar to men, seminomas are typically identified in bilaterally affected testicles. Primary testicular tumors include seminomas, Sertoli cell, and interstitial cell (Leydig) tumors. Rarely reported testicular tumors arising from other cell lineages include hemangiomas, granulose cell tumors, teratomas, sarcomas, embryonal carcinomas, gonadoblastomas, lymphomas, and rete testis mucinous adenocarcinomas.

Cryptorchidism appears to influence the age at which tumors develop, tumor incidence, and tumor type. In one study, all of the testicular tumors that developed from abdominal cryptorchids were identified before 10 years of age, suggesting that cryptorchidism speeds up testicular tumorigenesis in canines. Retained testes or testicles that were retained at some point are at a 9–14.3 times greater risk of developing neoplasia compared to testicles that descended normally. Interstitial cell tumors (43.2%) and seminomas (31.8%) are most common in scrotal testes, while Sertoli cell tumors accounted for only 11.4% of canine intra-scrotal neoplasms. By comparison, in cryptorchid testes seminoma (36.5%), mixed tumors (30.7%),

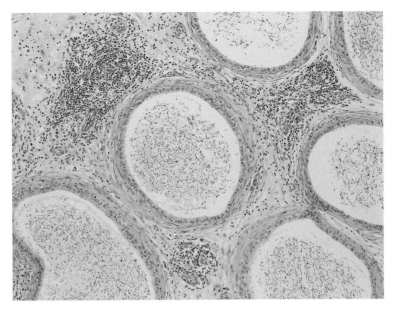

Figure 4.11 Chronic epididymitis. The epididymal interstitium is moderately expanded by loose fibrous connective tissue multifocally infiltrated by moderate to numerous lymphocytes and plasma cells.

and sertoli cell tumors (21.3%) are the most common and interstitial cell tumors (11.5%) the least. The occurrence rate of Sertoli cell tumors and seminomas is much higher in cryptorchid canine testes compared to scrotal testes.

Primary testicular tumors are histologically classified into germ cell tumors and sex cord-stromal tumors (Sertoli cell tumors, granulosa cell tumors, and Leydig cell tumors).

Sertoli Cell Tumors

Sertoli cell tumors are frequently associated with cryptorchidism or clinically with hormonal imbalance. Sertoli cell tumors can be subdivided by pattern into intratubular and diffuse, though both patterns are often present in the same testicle. Neoplastic cells are fusiform, often with extensive regions of palisading along the supporting stroma. Neoplastic cells have small, oval to elongate, often basally located nuclei with finely stippled chromatin and prominent nucleoli. Neoplastic cells have abundant, vacuolated to lightly eosinophilic cytoplasm and indistinct cytoplasmic boundaries. Tumor cells are typically supported on a moderate fibrous stroma, which helps to explain the very firm appearance that is typically identified on gross inspection (Figure 4.12a, b).

Seminoma

An association between cryptorchidism and seminomas has been reported in men, dogs, and horses. Seminomas are characterized by large, polyhedral to individualizing cells with a high nucleus to cytoplasmic ratio. Neoplastic cells have large, round vesiculate nuclei with prominent nucleoli. Anisokaryosis may be marked and high mitotic indices are common. Cells have scant to moderate amphophilic to basophilic cytoplasm and relatively distinct cytoplasmic boundaries. In poorly fixed specimens, cells may begin to individualize. Neoplastic cells exhibit invasive rather than expansive growth. Seminomas can be subdivided by pattern into intratubular and diffuse, though both patterns are often present in the same testicle, especially in more advanced tumors (Figures 4.13a, b and 4.14).

Interstitial Cell (Leydig) Tumor

Interstitial Cell Tumors are similar in appearance to normal testicular interstitial cells. They are polyhedral, arranged in solid sheets and, unlike Sertoli cell tumors, generally have minimal supporting stroma. Neoplastic cells have small, round to irregular nuclei with finely stippled chromatin and prominent nucleoli. Anisokaryosis is typically mild and mitotic figures rare. Neoplastic cells have abundant cytoplasm, which may vary from diffusely granular and eosinophilic, to vacuolated with well-demarcated lipid vacuoles (Figure 4.15a, b).

(a) 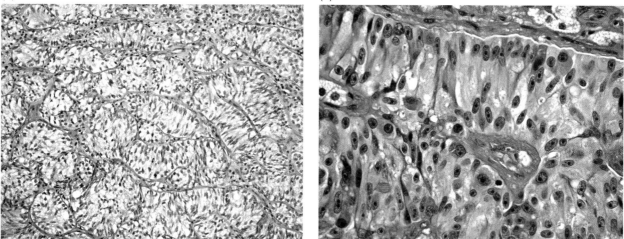 (b)

Figure 4.12   (a, b) Sertoli cell tumor. The tumor is composed of a uniform proliferation of fusiform cells arranged in irregular tubular structures separated by fine to moderate fibrovascular trabeculae. Fusiform cells are often oriented perpendicular to the basal lamina, have moderately-sized, oval, often basally located nuclei and abundant eosinophilic cytoplasm.

(a) 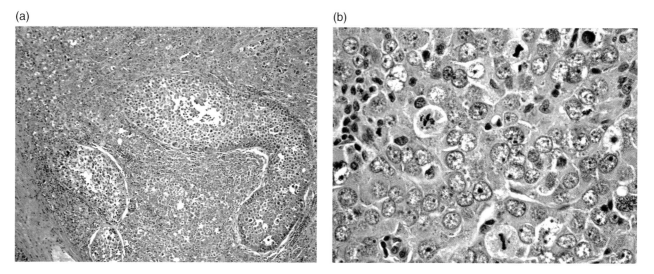 (b)

Figure 4.13   (a, b) Seminoma. The tumor is composed of a uniform population of polyhedral to individualizing cells with a high nucleus to cytoplasmic ratio arranged in solid sheets within tubular structures or infiltrating the interstitium. Neoplastic cells have large, round vesiculate nuclei with prominent nucleoli. Anisokaryosis is marked, and there are numerous mitotic figures. Cells have scant to moderate amphiphilic to basophilic cytoplasm and relatively distinct cytoplasmic boundaries.

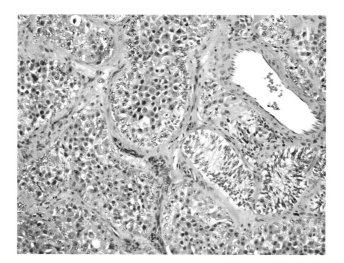

Figure 4.14   Sertoli cell tumor and seminoma. Testicle containing both a seminoma (polyhedral to individualizing cells) and a Sertoli cell tumor (fusiform cells).

(a)　　　　　　　　　　　　　　　　　　　　(b)

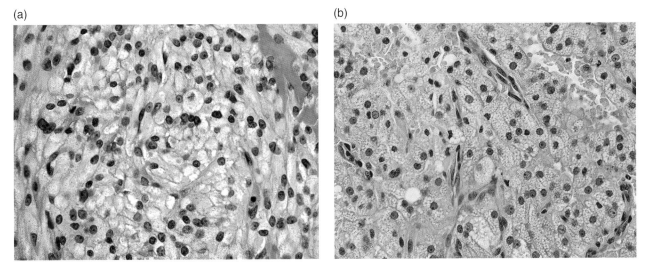

Figure 4.15　(a, b) Interstitial (Leydig) cell tumor. The tumor is composed of a uniform population of polyhedral cells arranged in solid sheets. Neoplastic cells have small, round to irregular nuclei with finely stippled chromatin and prominent nucleoli. Anisokaryosis is mild and mitotic figures rare. Neoplastic cells have abundant diffusely granular eosinophilic cytoplasm (left), which may contain well-demarcated lipid vacuoles (right).

Biologic Behavior of Canine Testicular Tumors

For all of the primary testicular tumors, the small number of animals with documented metastasis confirms that in dogs these tumors have a predominantly benign biological behavior, and castration is typically expected to be curative. Seminomas are the most malignant appearing of the testicular tumors, yet these have a reported metastatic rate of <10%.

Feline Testicular Tumors

Testicular tumors are rare in cats, but seminomas, interstitial cell tumors, Sertoli cell tumors, mixed tumors, and teratomas have all been reported.

Equine Testicular Tumors

In equines, neoplasms of male reproductive tract are most commonly detected in the testes, penis, and prepuce. In the horse, three neoplasms have been associated with cryptorchidism, including interstitial cell tumors, teratomas, and seminomas. In younger males, teratomas are the most common testicular neoplasm, whereas seminomas are the most commonly reported testicular tumor of the mature stallion. Interstitial (Leydig) cell and mixed germ cell stromal tumors have also been reported. Sertoli cell tumors are uncommon, 50% occur in cryptorchid testes, and in the limited reports available, 50% metastasized widely.

Though reports describing the biologic behavior of equine testicular tumors are limited, testicular tumors in equines tend to exhibit more aggressive biologic behavior. Abdominal testicular teratomas, teratocarcinomas, and embryonal carcinomas may metastasize and implant throughout the abdomen in young horses. Large seminomas are commonly malignant, may metastasize widely, and implant on peritoneal surfaces.

Penis and Prepuce

Introduction

The penis functions as a shared outlet for the elimination of urine and the deposition of spermatozoa into the female reproductive tract. Nonetheless, it is the copulatory function that is the main driving force behind penile anatomy. Much of the penis consists of erectile tissue, which varies from vascular (canine, equine, feline) to fibrous (swine, ruminants). The prepuce is a tubular sheath of skin attached to the ventral body wall that covers the free part of the nonerect penis.

Developmental and Degenerative Diseases

It is uncommon for the surgical pathologist to receive samples from developmental diseases of the penis and prepuce. The most common anomalies are phimosis (small preputial opening preventing protrusion of the penis), paraphimosis (inversion of the preputial opening forming a constrictive ring after penile protrusion preventing return of the penis into the preputial cavity), and a persistent frenulum. Penile and preputial hypoplasia may result from early castration or intersex abnormalities.

Inflammatory Diseases

Balanitis, Posthitis and Balanoposthitis

Balanitis (inflammation of the glans penis), posthitis (inflammation or the prepuce), and balanoposthitis (inflammation of the penis and prepuce) have been reported in all species. Because a large number and variety of organisms normally colonize the preputial cavity, some inflammation, including nodular lymphoid follicles, is to be expected. Pathologic inflammation may result from infectious agents, postpuberal alterations in immunity, the presence of foreign bodies, or trauma. Of special interest are contagious pathogens, such as herpesviruses in cattle, horses, and goats, which cause pustular, necrotizing, and ulcerative lesions of the penis.

A review of surgical pathology submissions at our institution showed that biopsies of non-neoplastic lesions of the penis and prepuce were most commonly submitted from horses, with "summer sores" or cutaneous habronemiasis. Habronemiasis results from the deposition of *Draschia megastoma* and *Habronema* sp. eggs in wounds and moist mucosa of the prepuce and penis and is typically observed during the summer months. Ulcerated lesions and single or multiple nodules that have draining tracks are common with this seasonal disease. The parasites induce deep, eosinophilic, fibrosing, granulomatous, and fistulating lesions in the prepuce, penis, and urethral process. These granulomas may be large enough to lead to penile prolapse. Small eosinophilic abscesses may surround intact or dead larvae, but larvae are not always seen. Habronemiasis may coexist in ulcerated neoplastic lesions (Figure 4.16a, b).

Neoplastic Diseases

Equine Penile Neoplasia

Penile and preputial neoplasia is more prevalent in equines than in other domestic animals, accounting for 6–10% of all neoplasms in the horse. SCC is the most common penile and preputial neoplasm. In addition, sarcoids, squamous papillomas, melanomas, fibromas, fibrosarcoma, lymphoma, and hemangiomas have all been reported.

(a)   (b)

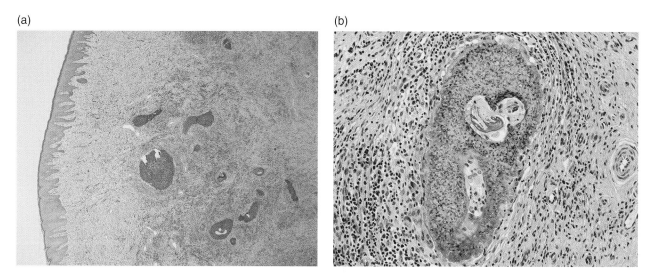

Figure 4.16   (a, b) Equine penile habronemiasis. There are multifocal, eosinophilic, fibrosing, and granulomatous lesions in the penile submucosa (left), which multifocally contain central, degenerate and mineralizing nematode larvae (right).

Equine Penile Squamous Cell Carcinoma

SCCs are the most common neoplasm involving the penis, prepuce, or both. Adult horses, especially horses with unpigmented skin, are most commonly affected. Epidemiologic, clinical, and experimental data support a causative role for both solar damage and *Equus caballus* papillomavirus type 2, which has been identified in equine genital SCC and precursor lesions. SCC develops as locally extensive to multicentric lesions. The lesion can be deep and ulcerated, multifocal and plaque-like, or exophytic with a papilliferous surface. Often, early lesions have solar keratosis or focal, epidermal anaplasia of carcinoma in situ. The neoplasms grow to disrupt the basement membrane with proliferating, anaplastic keratinocytes with dyskeratosis, numerous mitoses, and accompanying fibroplasia. SCCs of the penis and prepuce are locally invasive and recur locally in 17–25% of cases. These tumors have somewhat limited metastatic potential as only 16% of genital SCCs were metastatic, typically to regional lymph nodes (Figure 4.17).

Equine Penile Sarcoid

Equine sarcoids may occur on the equine penis and prepuce. These are locally aggressive, fibroblastic skin tumors, which can appear as either singular or multiple, flat or cauliflower-like growths, usually in young horses. Sarcoids have been clinically categorized into several groups including verrucous, fibroblastic, mixed verrucous and fibroblastic, occult, nodular, and malevolent.

Equine Penile Melanoma

Melanoma is a common, generally slow-growing, locally invasive tumor, estimated to occur in approximately 80% of aging gray horses. Equine melanocytic tumors can occur on the penis and prepuce and have been divided into four separate forms based on their distinct clinical, histological, and behavioral characteristics. These include melanocytic nevus, dermal melanoma, dermal melanomatosis, and anaplastic melanoma.

Melanocytic nevi occur in young horses of all coat colors and are benign, generally solitary, discrete, superficial masses. Melanocytic nevi (melanocytoma) are located in the superficial dermis or dermoepidermal junction. There is frequent epithelial involvement with distinct nests of relatively large, frequently mildly to moderately pleomorphic, epithelioid to spindle-shaped tumor cells with euchromatic nuclei, occasional binucleate cells, variable cytoplasmic pigmentation, and occasional mitoses. Complete surgical excision is generally curative.

Dermal melanomas occur as discrete tumor masses in gray horses. These tumors are generally single masses, but they may be multiple. Dermal melanomas have a deep dermal location with small, homogenous, indistinct, round, or dendritic tumor cells with condensed chromatin and dense cytoplasmic pigmentation and no visible mitoses. Similar to melanocytic nevi, complete surgical excision is typically curative.

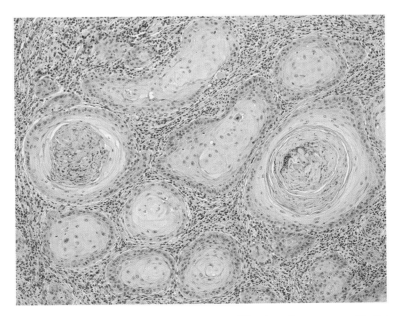

Figure 4.17 Equine penile SCC. The tumor is composed of an invasive proliferation of squamous epithelial cells arranged in clusters that often surround central laminations of keratin.

Dermal melanomatosis occurs in older gray horses, usually over 15 years of age, and most frequently involves the ventral tail, perineum, and external genitalia. Horses with dermal melanomatosis have multiple, frequently confluent masses with cellular features indistinguishable from those of dermal melanomas. Surgical excision of melanomatosis is generally not feasible, and these tumors have a high metastatic rate.

Anaplastic melanomas are composed of sheets of extremely pleomorphic epithelioid cells, with single-cell epithelial invasion, poor pigmentation, and numerous mitoses. Dermal melanomatosis and anaplastic melanoma represent the most invasive and metastatic melanocytic tumors in the horse.

Bovine Penile Fibropapilloma

Bovine fibropapillomas are benign, transmissible tumors that typically affect the penis of young bulls and are induced by papillomavirus infection. Tumors may be sessile or nodular early in their development and may grow to become large ulcerated, fungoid masses. The two most frequent sites are the junction of the glans penis and sheath and the craniodorsal part of the penis, which is prone to trauma. Ulceration and hemorrhage are frequent, particularly in large tumors. Because these tumors are virally induced, spontaneous regression is common. Tumors are composed mainly of interlacing streams and bundles of spindle cells, which may be plump and have frequent mitotic figures. Spindle cells often have large bizarre nucleoli. There is typically marked proliferation of the associated surface epithelium similar to pseudoepitheliomatous hyperplasia. If biopsy material is limited, rapidly growing fibropapillomas may have the appearance of fibrosarcomas (Figure 4.18).

Canine Penile Papilloma

Squamous papillomas of the canine penis and prepuce may be induced by canine papillomavirus, develop spontaneously, or arise following local trauma or irritation. Rarely these tumors can develop into squamous cell carcinomas. They may have a plaque-like or more typical raised papillomatous appearance. Microscopic changes are characteristic of a squamous papilloma at any location and consist of papillary hyperplasia of the epithelium of the penis or prepuce that is supported by a scant to moderate connective-tissue stroma (Figure 4.19).

Canine Transmissible Venereal Tumor

The canine transmissible venereal tumor (CTVT) has been reported worldwide but is uncommon in North and Central Europe and North America, mainly because of efforts to control stray dog populations. The disease usually (80%) occurs in dogs of reproductive age (two to eight years old) and less often in older animals. CTVT is a transmissible tumor where neoplastic cells are transferred from one host to another, typically during coitus. An intact epithelial barrier prevents

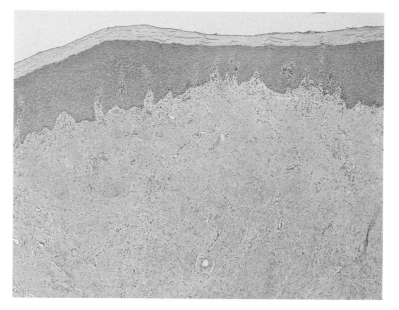

Figure 4.18   Bovine penile fibropapilloma. The tumor is composed of a moderately hyperplastic overlying penile epithelium above proliferating plump spindle cells arranged in interlacing streams and bundles supported on a moderate collagenous stroma.

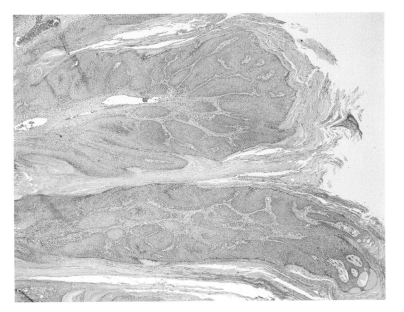

Figure 4.19 Canine penile papilloma. The exophytic penile mass is composed of multiple papillary projections of well-differentiated stratified squamous epithelium, supported on moderate fibrovascular stroma and covered by moderate, ortho, and parakeratotic hyperkeratosis with scattered serocellular surface crusts.

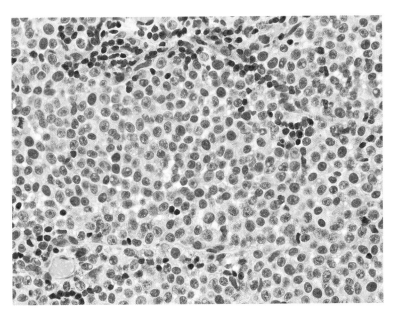

Figure 4.20 Transmissible venereal tumor. The tumor is composed of a uniform population of individual round cells arranged in solid sheets. Individual round cells have relatively well-defined cell borders, moderate to abundant, eosinophilic cytoplasm, and large, centrally located nuclei with finely stippled to coarse chromatin and a single prominent nucleolus. Low numbers of lymphocytes have multifocally infiltrated the round cell population.

natural transmission, which requires an abraded mucosa for the tumor to become established. In male dogs, neoplastic lesions are located on the more caudal part (bulbus glandis, 81.5%) and less often on the shaft (pars longa glandis, 25.9%) or the tip (9.9%) of the glans penis. The tumor is cauliflower-like, pedunculated, nodular, papillary, or multilobular and may be solitary or multifocal. In most dogs, CTVT undergoes a predictable cycle which includes an initial growth phase lasting four to six months, a stable phase, and a regression phase. CTVTs are antigenic, and the course of the disease is influenced by the host's immune status. Regressing tumors contain higher numbers of lymphocytes. In healthy, immuno-competent, adult dogs, the tumor regresses spontaneously after a period of months and immunity prevents successive occurrences, although not all tumors will regress. Metastasis is uncommon (5%). When it occurs, it is usually to the regional lymph nodes including inguinal and external iliac lymph nodes, but it is occasionally widespread.

Histologically, transmissible venereal tumors can be difficult to distinguish from other round cell tumors such as histiocytomas or lymphosarcoma. CTVT is typically unencapsulated and highly cellular, composed of dense sheets of round to polygonal cells separated by fine fibrovascular stroma. Cells have relatively well-defined cell borders, moderate to abundant, eosinophilic cytoplasm, which may be finely vacuolated, and large, centrally located nuclei with finely stippled to coarse chromatin and generally a single prominent nucleolus. Anisocytosis and anisokaryosis are typically mild, but tumors often have a high mitotic index. Multifocally, lymphocytes, plasma cells, and eosinophils may be scattered among the neoplastic cells. CTVT's stain with antibodies against vimentin, lysozyme, α-1-antitrypsin, and glial fibrillary acidic protein and are negative for keratins, S100, and muscle markers (Figure 4.20).

References and Additional Readings

Bell, F.W., Klausner, J.S., Hayden, D.W. et al. (1991). Clinical and pathologic features of prostatic adenocarcinoma in sexually intact and castrated dogs: 31 cases (1970–1987). *J. Am. Vet. Med. Assoc.* 199: 1623–1630.

Bhanmeechao, C., Srisuwatanasagul, S., and Ponglowhapan, S. (2018). Age-related changes in interstitial fibrosis and germ cell degeneration of the canine testis. *Reprod. Domest. Anim.* 53 (Suppl 3): 37–43.

Brinsko, S.P. (1998). Neoplasia of the male reproductive tract. *Vet. Clin. North Am. Equine Pract.* 14 (3): 517–533.

Camargo-Castañeda, A.M., Stranahan, L.W., Edwards, J.F. et al. (2021). Characterization of epididymal and testicular histologic lesions and use of immunohistochemistry and PCR on formalin-fixed tissues to detect *Brucella canis* in male dogs. *J. Vet. Diagn. Investig.* 33 (2): 352–356.

Christensen, B.W. (2018). Canine prostate disease. *Vet. Clin. North Am. Small Anim. Pract.* 48 (4): 701–719.

Foster, R.A. (2012). Common lesions in the male reproductive tract of cats and dogs. *Vet. Clin. North Am. Small Anim. Pract.* 42 (3): 527–545.

Ganguly, B., Das, U., and Das, A.K. (2016). Canine transmissible venereal tumour: a review. *Vet. Comp. Oncol.* 14 (1): 1–12.

Hall, W.C., Nielsen, S.W., and McEntee, K. (1976). Tumours of the prostate and penis. *Bull. World Health Organ.* 53 (2–3): 247–256.

Hesser, A.C. and Davidson, A.P. (2015). Spermatocele in a South African Boerboel dog. *Top Companion Anim. Med.* 30 (1): 28–30.

Johnston, S.D., Kamolpatana, K., Root-Kustritz, M.V. et al. (2000). Prostatic disorders in the dog. *Anim. Reprod. Sci.* 60–61: 405–415.

Lai, C., van den Ham, R., van Leenders, G. et al. (2008). Histopathological and immunohistochemical characterization of canine prostate cancer. *Prostate* 68: 477–488.

Liao, A.T., Chu, P.Y., Yeh, L.S. et al. (2009). A 12-year retrospective study of canine testicular tumors. *J. Vet. Med. Sci.* 71 (7): 919–923.

Manuali, E., Forte, C., Porcellato, I. et al. (2020). A five-year cohort study on testicular tumors from a population-based canine cancer registry in Central Italy (Umbria). *Prev. Vet. Med.* 185 (105201).

Miller, M.A., Hartnett, S.E., and Ramos-Vara, J.A. (2007). Interstitial cell tumor and Sertoli cell tumor in the testis of a cat. *Vet. Pathol.* 44 (3): 394–397.

Nieto, J.M., Pizarro, M., Balaguer, L.M. et al. (1989). Canine testicular tumors in descended and cryptorchid testes. *Dtsch. Tierarztl. Wochenschr.* 96 (4): 186–189.

Palmieri, C., Lean, F.Z., Akter, S.H. et al. (2014). A retrospective analysis of 111 canine prostatic samples: histopathological findings and classification. *Res. Vet. Sci.* 97 (3): 568–573.

Palmieri, C., Foster, R.A., Grieco, V. et al. (2019). Histopathological terminology standards for the reporting of prostatic epithelial lesions in dogs. *J. Comp. Pathol.* 171: 30–37.

Pecile, A., Groppetti, D., Pizzi, G. et al. (2021). Immunohistochemical insights into a hidden pathology: canine cryptorchidism. *Theriogenology* 176: 43–53.

Pratt, S.M., Stacy, B.A., Whitcomb, M.B. et al. (2003). Malignant Sertoli cell tumor in the retained abdominal testis of a unilaterally cryptorchid horse. *J. Am. Vet. Med. Assoc.* 222 (4): 486–490.

Pusterla, N., Watson, J.L., Wilson, W.D. et al. (2003). Cutaneous and ocular habronemiasis in horses: 63 cases (1988–2002). *J. Am. Vet. Med. Assoc.* 222 (7): 978–982.

Rizk, A., Mosbah, E., Karrouf, G. et al. (2013). Surgical management of penile and preputial neoplasms in equine with special reference to partial phallectomy. *J. Vet. Med.* 2013: 891413.

Smith, J. (2008). Canine prostatic disease: a review of anatomy, pathology, diagnosis, and treatment. *Theriogenology* 70 (3): 375–383.

Valentine, B.A. (1995). Equine melanocytic tumors: a retrospective study of 53 horses (1988 to 1991). *J. Vet. Intern. Med.* 9 (5): 291–297.

Van Den Top, J.G., Ensink, J.M., Gröne, A. et al. (2010). Penile and preputial tumours in the horse: literature review and proposal of a standardized approach. *Equine Vet. J.* 42 (8): 746–757.

Zirkin, B.R. and Strandberg, J.D. (1984). Quantitative changes in the morphology of the aging canine prostate. *Anat. Rec.* 208: 207–214.

5

Pathology of the Female Reproductive System

Michael J. Yaeger

Department of Veterinary Pathology, Iowa State University, Ames, IA, USA

Ovaries

Introduction

The two main functions of the ovary are the production of hormones and ova. The ovary is surrounded by a dense connective tissue capsule, the tunica albuginea, and is divided into a cortex and medulla. The cortex is composed of a loose stroma surrounding corpora lutei and follicles in various stages of development. Except in the horse, the medulla is centrally located and consists primarily of loose connective tissue, blood vessels, lymphatics, and the rete ovary, which are tubular channels of epithelial cells. The histological appearance of the ovary varies considerably between species, and it is important to recognize unique features in each species to prevent inappropriate interpretation.

Developmental and Degenerative Diseases

A variety of forms of intersexuality have been described in domestic animals, and only a brief mention will be made of these abnormalities. Perhaps the most economically important intersex is the freemartin, a condition most commonly reported in cattle but which has also been recognized in sheep, goats, and swine. The bovine freemartin is an infertile female twin of a normal bull. The gonads of the freemartin are a mixture of male and female elements, although the distribution of these elements is variable. Masculinized female gonads are termed ovotestes. The tubular genital tract is usually incompletely developed, and male secondary sex glands are present (Figure 5.1).

The ovary of the bitch is characterized by the presence of cords and nests of cells beneath the surface epithelium, the so-called subsurface epithelial structures that arise from the surface epithelium. These proliferations are very prominent at certain stages of development in the fetal ovary and increase in number and prominence with advancing age. Hyperplasia and cystic dilation of these structures can occur, usually in geriatric bitches. Cystic dilatation and/or hyperplasia of the rete ovarii also occurs with advancing age.

Ovarian Cysts
Cysts occurring within the ovary include follicular cysts, luteal cysts (luteinized follicular cyst), cystic corpora lutea, cystic rete ovarii, inclusion cysts derived from the surface epithelium, and cysts of the subsurface epithelial structures. Luteal and follicular cysts are derived from anovulatory Graafian follicles and likely represent different manifestations of the same condition. They are most common in the cow and the sow, although they do occur in other species and usually interfere with normal reproductive function in nonpregnant animals.

Anovulatory follicles continue to enlarge, so cystic follicles are, at least initially, larger than normal tertiary follicles. Follicular cysts in the sow are frequently multiple and usually have areas of luteinization in the wall. The thickness of the granulosa cell layer that forms the lining of follicular cysts varies considerably between cysts, as does the extent of luteinization of the theca and granulosa cell layers. Luteinization is far more extensive in luteal cysts than it is in

Atlas of Veterinary Surgical Pathology, First Edition. Edited by Joseph S. Haynes.
© 2023 John Wiley & Sons, Inc. Published 2023 by John Wiley & Sons, Inc.

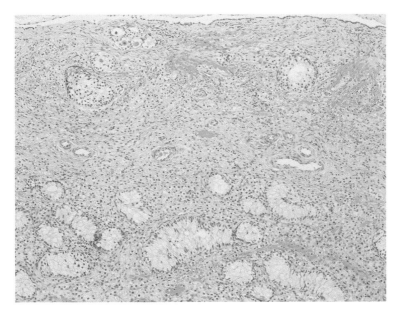

Figure 5.1   Ovotestes. The gonadal tissue consists of primitive seminiferous tubules (lower aspect of photo) and developing follicular structures (upper portion of photo).

follicular cysts; however, the degree of luteinization required to justify classification as a luteal cyst compared to a follicular cyst has not been well defined. In both types of cysts, an ovum is not usually found in the antrum.

Cystic corpora lutea are merely normal corpora lutea with a central cavity and do not cause functional problems. They are distinguished from anovulatory follicular cysts because they derive from follicles from which ovulation has occurred and therefore have an ovulation papilla. Cystic corpora lutea apparently produce sufficient progesterone in pregnant animals to maintain pregnancy and occur in a variety of animal species.

Cysts of the surface epithelium occur relatively commonly in the mare and bitch. In the bitch, they usually derive from the subsurface epithelial structures. In the mare, cysts of the surface epithelium may become extensive and interfere with reproductive function. Cysts of the surface epithelium and subsurface epithelial structures are often multiple and remain confined to the ovarian cortex. The cysts are lined by cuboidal epithelium (Figure 5.2).

Cystic rete ovarii are most common in the bitch and the queen. The rete ovarii are normally located in the hilus of the ovary. Cystic rete ovarii appear as dilated epithelial-lined tubules, which can become large enough to compress the cortex of the affected ovary (Figure 5.3).

Ovarian Inflammation

Oophoritis and Salpingitis

Infectious diseases that involve the ovaries of domestic animals appear to be uncommon, due in part to the routine removal of the uterus and ovaries in dogs and cats at an early age. Infectious agents can reach the ovary hematogenously, or as an extension from either peritonitis or salpingitis. Granulomatous oophoritis can occur in animals that have either tuberculosis or brucellosis, although the incidence of these two diseases has now been greatly reduced in many countries. Pyogenic infections of the ovary and its surrounding tissues occur sporadically due to *Trueperella pyogenes* in cattle and swine and *Corynebacterium pseudotuberculosis* (caseous lymphadenitis) in sheep.

Ovarian Neoplasia

Tumors of the ovary have been described in all the domestic species, although they are relatively uncommon. The common practice of spaying female pets, the abbreviated lifespan of many production animal species, and overlooking small tumors because ovaries are often not routinely examined, may all contribute to this apparent low prevalence. Classification of primary ovarian tumors is based on the assumption that these tumors arise from one of three ovarian components: germ cells, the ovarian stroma, or the epithelium, either of the ovarian surface or rete ovarii.

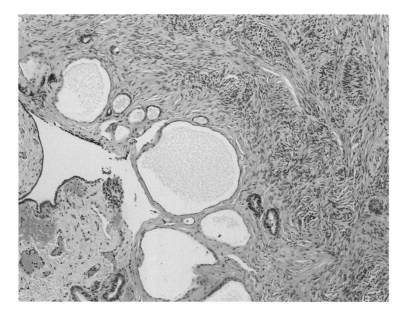

Figure 5.2 Ovarian subsurface epithelial cysts. Directly beneath the ovarian surface are multiple, variably-size cystic structures filled with clear fluid and lined by a well-differentiated, simple, flattened to cuboidal epithelium.

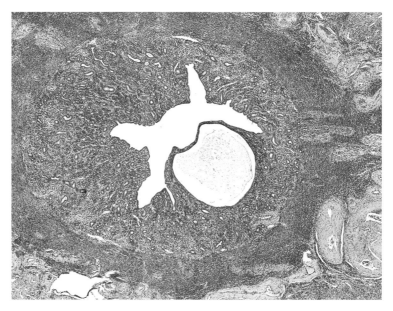

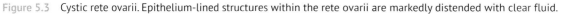

Figure 5.3 Cystic rete ovarii. Epithelium-lined structures within the rete ovarii are markedly distended with clear fluid.

Germ Cell Tumors/Dysgerminoma and Teratoma

Dysgerminomas and teratomas are derived from germ cells, and both occur in domestic animals.

Dysgerminoma

Dysgerminomas are essentially the female equivalent of testicular seminomas. These are rare in domestic animals but have been reported in most species, most commonly the bitch and queen. Dysgerminomas are highly cellular tumors, consisting of broadsheets, cords, and nests of large, individual, polyhedral cells separated by connective tissue septa. Cells have vesicular nuclei and prominent nucleoli. Multinucleate cells and focal aggregations of lymphocytes may be present. Metastasis can occur. Hypertrophic osteopathy has been described in mares with dysgerminomas (Figure 5.4).

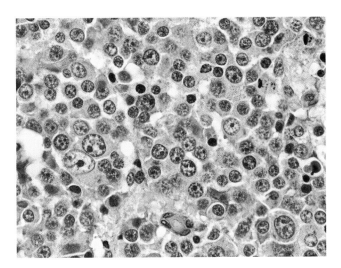

Figure 5.4   Dysgerminoma. The tumor is composed of a solid sheet of large, individual, polyhedral cells with vesicular nuclei, prominent nucleoli, scant to moderate eosinophilic cytoplasm, marked anisokaryosis, and anisocytosis.

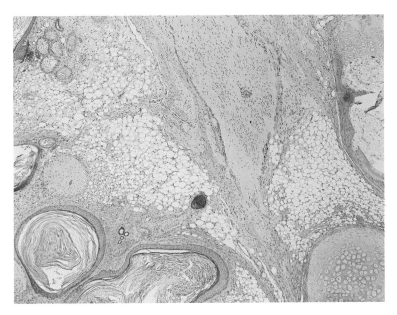

Figure 5.5   Ovarian teratoma. The tumor consists of well-differentiated nervous and adipose tissue, islands of hyaline cartilage, clusters of cells exhibiting sebaceous differentiation, a developing hair follicle, and keratin-filled, stratified squamous epithelium-lined cystic structures.

Teratoma

Teratomas are composed of tissue derived from at least two, and often all three, germinal layers. Presumably, they arise from pluripotential stem cells. Ovarian teratomas are uncommon in domestic animals but have been described in most species. They typically have solid and cystic areas, the latter often containing sebaceous material or hair. A variety of other tissue types may be present, including bone, cartilage, teeth, and nervous tissue. Malignant teratomas have been described, particularly in the bitch (Figure 5.5).

Sex Cord-Stromal Tumors

Sex cord-stromal tumors are derived from, or histologically resemble, the normal cellular constituents of the ovary other than epithelium or germ cells. The term "sex cord-stromal" reflects the uncertain origin of these tumors, which have been variously designated as granulosa cell tumors, luteomas, thecomas, Sertoli cell tumors of the ovary, Leydig cell tumors,

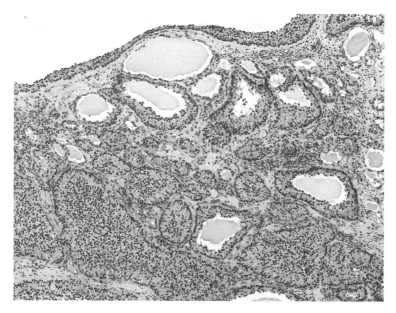

Figure 5.6   Granulosa cell tumor. This sex cord-stromal tumor is composed of granulosa cells arranged in solid clusters or cystic structures resembling developing follicles.

androblastoma, arrhenoblastoma, or lipid cell tumors. Sex cord-stromal tumors share the potential to be hormonally active and to secrete a diverse mixture of male and female sex hormones, which may impact the animal's reproductive behavior leading to prolonged anestrus, nymphomania, or masculinization. Hormones produced by these tumors can also induce changes in extraovarian tissues, especially the tubular genital tract.

With the probable exception of the sow, sex cord-stromal tumors are the most common form of ovarian neoplasm in all species. In the bitch, sex cord-stromal tumors and tumors of the subsurface epithelial structures have a similar incidence. Sex cord-stromal tumors typically are polycystic and histologically are seen to consist of cysts that resemble disorganized attempts at follicle formation, accompanied by a prominent supporting stroma of spindle cells interpreted as theca cells. Within the follicular structures are multiple layers of cells that resemble granulosa cells, often with palisading at the periphery. In other tumors, the follicular pattern is less apparent, and neoplastic cells are arranged in solid cords and nests (Figure 5.6).

Epithelial Tumors

Epithelial tumors have been described in the mare, sow, queen, and cow but are uncommon in all domestic species except the bitch. The vast majority of epithelial tumors arise from the surface epithelium, although rarely, they arise from the rete ovarii. In the bitch, these tumors arise most frequently from the subsurface epithelial structures, which are themselves derived from the surface epithelium. Hyperplasia of the subsurface epithelial structures is very common in older bitches, and the distinction between hyperplasia and adenomas may be difficult.

Epithelial tumors of the ovary are usually cystic and papillary; thus, the names cystadenoma and cystadenocarcinoma are frequently used. Histologically, these tumors consist of arboriform papillae that project into the cyst lumen. The papillae consist of a connective tissue stalk that is lined by single or multiple layers of cuboidal or columnar epithelial cells that may or may not be ciliated. The wall of the cyst typically is also lined by epithelium, and the lumen of the cyst may contain proteinaceous material. In the absence of metastasis or obvious vascular invasion, malignant tumors are distinguished from benign adenomas by the presence of stromal invasion. The cyst wall, the connective tissue papillae, or the stroma of the adjacent ovary may be invaded. Metastasis of carcinomas tends to occur transcoelomically after rupture of cysts or invasion of the tumor through the capsule of the ovary and subsequent implantation in the abdominal cavity (Figures 5.7 and 5.8).

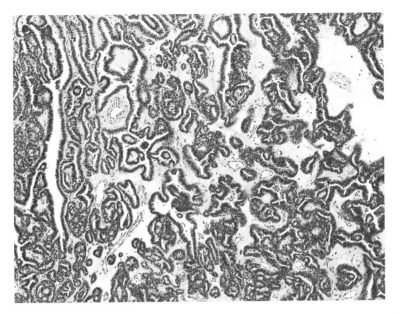

Figure 5.7   Ovarian cystadenoma. The tumor consists of arboriform papillae that project into cystic lumens. The papillae consist of a connective tissue stalk that is lined by a simple, columnar epithelium.

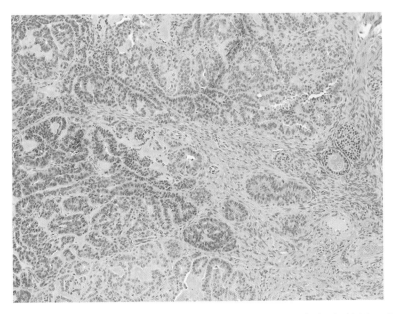

Figure 5.8   Ovarian adenocarcinoma. The tumor consists of arboriform papillae composed of cuboidal to columnar epithelial cells that have infiltrated into the ovarian stroma.

Uterus and Vagina

Introduction

The uterus accepts the fertilized ovum from the uterine tubes, provides fetal nourishment during gestation, and, along with the cervix and vagina, forms a passageway for birth of the fetus. Like all tissues in the female reproductive tract, the uterus and vagina undergo remarkable, hormone-induced cycle and pregnancy-related changes in their gross and microscopic appearances.

Developmental uterine anomalies are uncommon in cats and dogs but may be observed during elective ovariohysterectomy (OHE) or in cases of dystocia/retained fetuses. Aberrations in the development of the Müllerian duct can occur with varying degrees of severity, affecting uterine horn segments (segmental agenesis) or the entire uterine horn (unicornuate uterus). These anomalies have been detected in many domestic species, including cats, dogs, cows, horses, deer, sheep, pigs, ferrets, and alpacas. A common characteristic of segmental agenesis is the accumulation of fluid in the lumen of the affected uterine horn distal to the occlusion, which has the potential to result in hydrometra, mucometra, or pyometra. An association between uterine anomalies and renal agenesis has long been recognized in women. Because more than half of cats and dogs with uterine anomalies had ipsilateral renal agenesis, both kidneys should be assessed following the discovery of a unicornuate uterus or segmental uterine horn agenesis. Segmental uterine anomalies are typically not accompanied by ovarian hypoplasia/agenesis.

Uterine horns and the uterine body are composed of the endometrium, myometrium, and perimetrium, with endometrial glands in the endometrial layer and organized blood vessels in the myometrium and perimetrium. Uterine horns that lack a central lumen and endometrial layer and are composed of disorganized connective tissue, smooth muscle, and blood vessels are classified as unicornuate uterus. Similar changes involving a portion of the horn are classified as segmental agenesis.

Endometrial Hyperplasia/Cysts

Cystic uterine lesions can arise from the uterine serosa, myometrium, or endometrium and include: serosal inclusion cysts, adenomyosis, endometrial polyps, cystic remnants of mesonephric ducts, and cysts associated with endometrial hyperplasia. Endometrial cysts of the queen and bitch generally arise from endometrial glandular epithelium, unlike the mare, where most endometrial cysts are distensions of lymphatics, which is extremely rare in the bitch or queen. Although cystic endometrial hyperplasia (CEH) occurs in both the queen and bitch, it is much more common in the bitch, likely because of the longer periods during which the endometrium is under the influence of progesterone.

Serosal Inclusion Cysts

Serosal inclusion cysts are common and can become quite extensive. These are thin-walled structures found on the serosal surface of the uterus that may be single or form small, grape-like clusters. They develop along linear folds on the outer uterine surface from adhesions of the mesothelial serosal covering in older parous bitches, or in bitches that have had a cesarean operation. They are not found in queens. Cysts are lined by a single layer of flattened cuboidal epithelium and are present in the serosa or the deep layer of the myometrium.

Cystic Endometrial Hyperplasia

The complete pathogenesis of CEH is unclear and likely multifactorial. There is an undeniable hormone influence, particularly associated with progesterone, as 45% of bitches treated with medroxyprogesterone acetate developed CEH, whereas only 5% of untreated females had cystic lesions. There is also an association with age, likely reflecting repeated hormonal influence, as CEH was identified in 6.8% of two-year-old breeding bitches and 60.0% of six-year-old bitches. Histological changes in the endometrium with hyperplasia vary from mild to severe and include mild hyperplasia with thickening of the endometrium and elongation of the glands. As the glands continue to elongate, they become disorganized and convoluted with more prominent stroma. These glands then dilate, fill with secretion, and form variably-sized endometrial cysts (Figure 5.9).

Pseudoplacentational Endometrial Hyperplasia

A second form of endometrial cystic lesion occurs in a condition called pseudoplacentational endometrial hyperplasia. This lesion results from marked exuberant growth of the endometrium in either a diffuse or segmental pattern with marked resemblance to the maternal tissues beneath the normal canine zonary placenta. There is evidence that mild irritation, possibly associated with low-grade bacterial infection, is sufficient to initiate this proliferative chain of events but only when the endometrium is under the influence of progestogens. In this condition, partial fusion of thin villous folds arising from the superficial aspects of endometrial glands and folds arising from the luminal surface fuse to form cysts. Commonly there is coagulative necrosis of the luminal aspects of the endometrial folds that produce amorphic debris in the uterine lumen. Microscopically, the placenta-like zones have long branching villous structures, and the epithelial cells of the lumen and the glands are large and foamy. The endometrial glands are dilated and contain secretion.

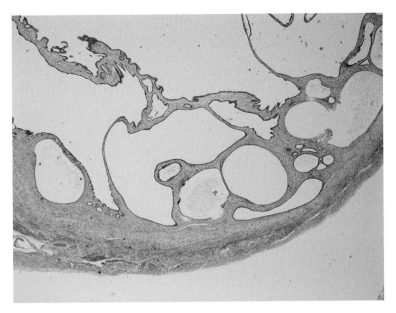

Figure 5.9 Canine cystic endometrial hyperplasia. The endometrium is markedly thickened by numerous variably-sized, cystically dilated endometrial glands.

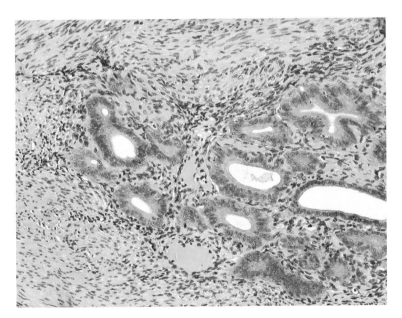

Figure 5.10 Uterine adenomyosis. The myometrial smooth muscle fibers are focally disrupted by small clusters of submucosal glands.

Adenomyosis

Adenomyosis is the presence of endometrial glands and stroma between the muscle bundles of the myometrium. These glands can become cystic, and if extensive, adenomyosis can produce a "Swiss cheese" appearance to the incised uterine wall. The presence of adenomyosis may weaken the uterine wall and is occasionally found at sites of uterine rupture in cases of pyometra (Figure 5.10).

Subinvolution of Placental Sites

Subinvolution of placental sites is a disorder of young, primiparous bitches that presents clinically as prolonged sanguineous vulvar discharge and is the result of delayed or complete failure of uterine involution after whelping. Studies suggest that normal involution of the genital tract in the bitch is slow and can take up to 12–15 weeks. Since subinvolution of

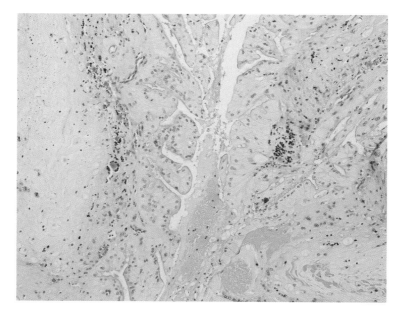

Figure 5.11   Canine placental subinvolution. The endometrium forms multiple papillary projections lined by large columnar epithelial cells with abundant, clear, foamy vacuolated cytoplasm and apically located vesicular nuclei. There is extensive luminal hemorrhage. The submucosa is expanded by an eosinophilic matrix with variable numbers of polygonal and multinucleated cells (trophoblasts).

placental sites looks histologically identical to normal involution, a good clinical history is essential for making an appropriate diagnosis. Consistent histological features include retention and invasion of trophoblast-like cells into the underlying stroma, the presence of large amounts of collagen at the placental site, extensive regions of necrosis and hemorrhage, and marked dilation of endometrial glands (Figure 5.11).

Uterine Inflammation

Endometritis, Metritis, Perimetritis, and Pyometra

Uterine inflammation can be broadly divided into several categories based on the extent of involvement of the uterine lumen and wall. Endometritis is an inflammatory reaction in the uterus limited to the endometrium. Metritis is an inflammatory reaction involving the entire uterine wall. Perimetritis is inflammation of the uterine serosa. Pyometra is suppurative inflammation of the uterus with an accumulation of pus in the lumen. Inflammation of the uterus is most commonly associated with bacterial infection. Early in uterine bacterial infection, there is a neutrophilic inflammatory infiltrate initially involving the superficial endometrium and surrounding endometrial glands, with neutrophils migrating through the surface and glandular epithelium. This is typically accompanied by vascular congestions and submucosal edema. In chronic endometritis, the composition of infiltrating inflammatory cells changes to include lymphocytes, plasma cells, and macrophages. Their distribution extends to the deeper endometrium and occasionally follows the stroma around blood vessels down into the myometrium. Chronic endometritis may also induce interstitial fibrosis (Figures 5.12 and 5.13).

Endometrial Biopsies

Endometrial biopsies are undertaken to gain prognostic information regarding the potential for future reproductive success and are a well-established procedure in human and equine medicine. The nature and severity of lesions are reflected in the category score or grade, and this score has been shown to correlate with reproductive outcomes, providing a useful tool in the diagnosis and treatment of subfertility in mares. The procedure has been used to a lesser extent in other species, including canines. Unfortunately, clinical follow-up on a sufficient number of canine cases to associate reproductive performance with histologic lesions is not yet available.

Endometrial biopsy sections are routinely stained with hematoxylin and eosin (H&E). Additionally, staining with Masson's trichrome can be used to highlight connective tissue and aid in the detection of fibrosis. Parameters assessed

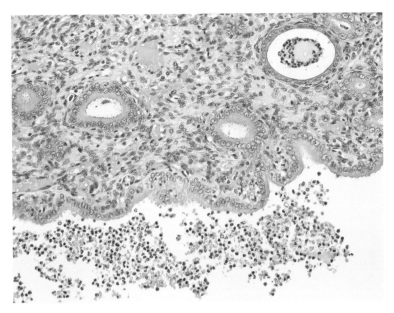

Figure 5.12 Pyometra. The uterine lumen is distended by an exudate composed of neutrophils and extravasated erythrocytes. Low numbers of neutrophils are present with the superficial submucosa, migrating through the surface epithelium and within mildly distended endometrial glands.

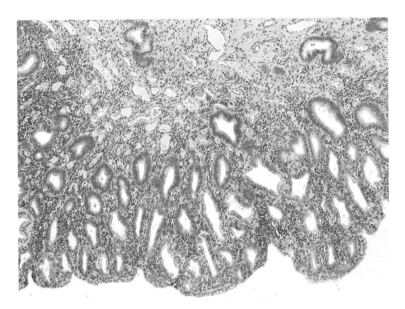

Figure 5.13 Chronic endometritis. The uterine submucosa is diffusely infiltrated by moderate numbers of lymphocytes and plasma cells.

during endometrial biopsy evaluation include (i) the luminal epithelium; (ii) fibrosis, (iii) inflammation, (iv) lymphatics (lymphatic lacunae), (v) the presence of infectious agents, and (vi) dilation of submucosal glands (bitch).

Similar to the mare, the most common reason for obtaining uterine biopsies in dogs is lack of conception. In one large canine endometrial biopsy study, the most prevalent lesion was endometritis (42.6% of cases), followed by cystic changes of the endometrium, including CEH (33.3% of cases), while in 27.8% of cases clinically relevant lesions that might explain the subfertility were not observed. Some degree of fibrosis was detected in 25.3% of dogs, including periglandular fibrosis (80.2%), interstitial fibrosis (10.9%), and fibrosis of the myometrium (13.9%). Uterine fibrosis was typically mild, even in cases of chronic endometritis, and it appears that this lesion is typically more subtle and less prevalent in the dog than in the mare.

Endometrial Fibrosis Endometrial fibrosis is considered to be a permanent or irreversible change. Fibrosis may involve isolated individual gland branches or surround a number of branches resulting in pathologic nesting of gland branches within a fibrotic matrix. Fibrosis is graded as mild (1–3 concentric layers), moderate (4–10 concentric layers), and severe (≥11 cell layers thick). Important locations for the assessment of stromal fibrosis include periglandular branching areas and the basement membrane of the luminal epithelium. Representative examples of common lesions described in endometrial biopsies including periglandular fibrosis, cystic glandular dilation, and glandular nesting are described below (Figure 5.14a–c).

Lymphatic Lacunae Lymphatic lacunae are dilated endometrial lymphatics and are most commonly observed in endometrial biopsies from mares. These may coalesce or enlarge to become endometrial cysts. Possible causes for lymphatic dysfunction may include large and pendulous uterine conformation; congenital malformations; infiltration or obstruction due to an inflammatory, fibrotic, or neoplastic process; and elevated lymphatic hydrostatic pressure from the impedance of flow (Figure 5.14d).

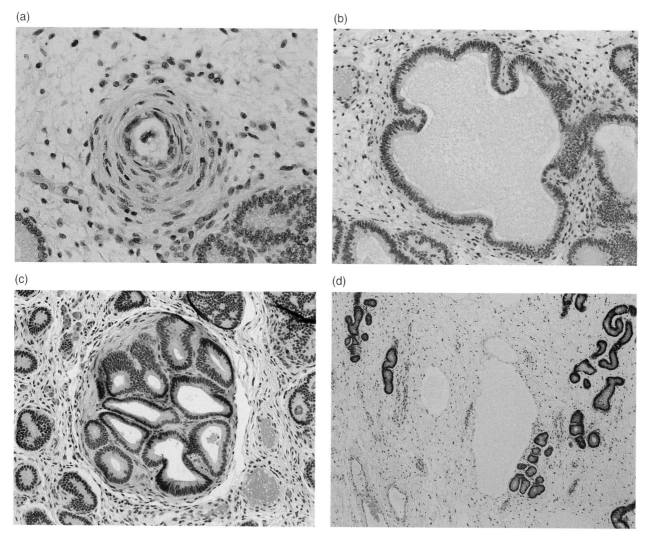

(a) (b) (c) (d)

Figure 5.14 (a) Endometrial periglandular fibrosis. Focally, the lumen of an endometrial gland is mildly dilated, lined by flattened (attenuated) epithelial cells, and surrounded by four to seven concentric layers of fibrous connective tissue. (b) Endometrial cystic glandular dilation. Focally, the lumen of an endometrial gland is markedly dilated, partially filled with amorphous eosinophilic fluid and surrounded by one to three concentric layers of fibrous connective tissue. (c) Endometrial glandular nesting. Multiple endometrial glands with moderately dilated lumens are clustered in close proximity by one to three concentric layers of fibrous connective tissue. (d) Endometrial lymphatic lacunae. Endometrial submucosal lymphatics are markedly dilated (lymphatic lacunae), and the adjacent stromal elements are moderately separated by clear spaces (edema).

Uterine and Vaginal Neoplasia

Endometrial Polyps

Endometrial polyps are focal tumor-like growths projecting into the uterine lumen and consist of endometrial glands and connective tissue stroma. Endometrial polyps have been detected in elderly bitches. Animals with endometrial polyps are often asymptomatic but can show mucopurulent or bloody vaginal discharge. Histologically, endometrial polyps consist of endometrial glands with varying degrees of cystic dilation and connective tissue stroma that may be edematous and hemorrhagic. There is no evidence that endometrial polyps in the dog are preneoplastic, and uterine cancer is uncommon in this species. These are more common in queens than in bitches. In other domestic animals, endometrial polyps are rare and considered benign (Figure 5.15).

Uterine Tumors

Benign and malignant tumors of the uterus typically arise from the endometrium or myometrium. In a study of 1489 female bovines at slaughter, there was a 0.4% ($n = 6$) incidence of uterine neoplasms, with 50% diagnosed as adenocarcinomas and the other 50% as leiomyomas. Bovine uterine adenocarcinomas are usually found in the uterine horns of 11–15-year-old cows, evoke a scirrhous response, and metastasize rapidly. Uterine adenocarcinomas are also the most common neoplasm in sexually intact female rabbits, and age appears to be the most important risk factor in its development. The incidence of uterine adenocarcinoma may be as high as 60% in rabbits >four years old and up to 80% in rabbits of certain breeds, such as Tan, French silver, Havana, and Dutch. Uterine adenocarcinomas in rabbits often develop as globular, polypoid masses and are generally multicentric and involve both uterine horns. Histologically, the tumors are well differentiated, may have necrotic or hemorrhagic centers, and may secrete mucus. Tumors usually grow slowly and eventually metastasize locally into the peritoneum, myometrium, local lymph nodes, and abdominal organs. Uterine tumors consist of 0.3–0.4% of all canine tumors. Leiomyomas and leiomyosarcomas are the most common, accounting for approximately 90 and 10%, respectively (Figures 5.16 and 5.17).

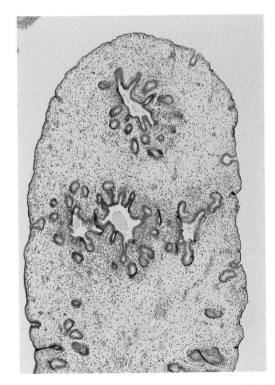

Figure 5.15 Canine endometrial polyp. The uterine mass consists of a focal papillary projection of the endometrium containing endometrial glands supported on an edematous stroma.

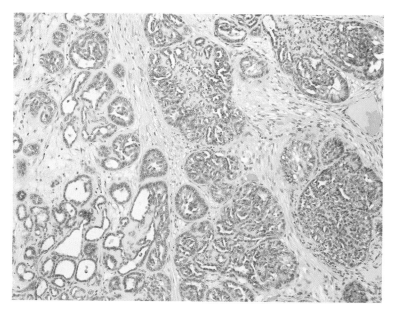

Figure 5.16   Rabbit uterine adenocarcinoma. The tumor is composed of an invasive population of epithelial cells forming multiple tubular structures lined by a cuboidal epithelium which frequently forms small papillary projections.

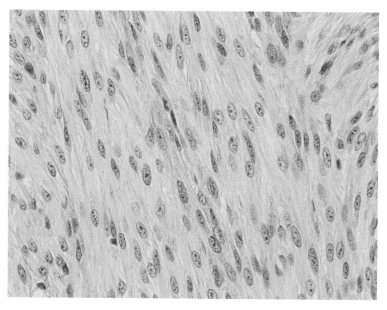

Figure 5.17   Uterine leiomyosarcoma. The tumor is composed of a uniform population of spindle cells arranges in streams. Spindle cells have large, oval vesiculate nuclei with multiple nucleoli. Spindle cells have moderate to abundant eosinophilic cytoplasm and indistinct cytoplasmic borders.

Vaginal and Vulvar Tumors

Vaginal and vulvar tumors are the second most common canine female reproductive tumor after those of the mammary gland. They constitute 2.4–3% of canine neoplasia. Nonmalignant vaginal and vulvar tumors reported in the veterinary literature include leiomyomas, fibroleiomyomas, fibromas, polyps, lipomas, sebaceous adenomas, fibrous histiocytomas, benign melanomas, myxomas, and myxofibromas. Malignant tumors reported to have arisen from the vaginal/vulvar region include transmissible venereal tumors, adenocarcinoma, squamous cell carcinoma, hemangiosarcoma, osteosarcoma, mast cell tumor, and epidermoid carcinoma.

Mammary Gland

Introduction

Mammary glands are large, compound tubuloalveolar glands. Each secretory unit, composed of an alveolus and associated secretory tubule, is surrounded by myoepithelial cells, which contract to force secretions into a system of ducts. The mammary gland epithelium is typically composed of a single layer of polarized luminal epithelial cells surrounded by a single outer layer of myoepithelial cells and scattered mammary stem cells able to generate both luminal and myoepithelial cells, all of which are separated from the intralobular stroma by a laminin-rich basement membrane. The mammary gland is hormonally responsive, with hormonal influence leading to physiologic or pathologic hyperplasia and contributing to mammary tumor development.

Developmental and Degenerative Diseases

Feline Mammary Fibroadenomatous Hyperplasia

The mammary gland is influenced by hormones and is susceptible to a variety of hyperplastic and dysplastic conditions. Feline mammary fibroadenomatous hyperplasia (fibroepithelial hyperplasia) is a progesterone-induced proliferation of the epithelium of mammary ducts and surrounding stroma that is manifest as marked, generalized enlargement of 1 or more mammary glands. The condition develops in young queens during early pregnancy, pseudopregnancy, or after receipt of progestogen injections. It can also develop in male cats treated with progesterone, particularly megestrol acetate. The condition typically occurs within one to two weeks after estrus or two to six weeks after progestin treatment. Histologically, there are branching and proliferation of mammary ducts lined by a simple columnar epithelium surrounded by massive and concentric proliferation of loose, edematous stroma (Figure 5.18).

Mammary Duct Ectasia and Hyperplasia

Mammary ectasia is cystic dilation of large mammary ducts, typically with accumulation of necrotic debris, variable numbers of foamy macrophages mixed with lipid material, and cholesterol clefts within duct lumens. Leakage of material from dilated ducts can lead to granulomatous inflammation in the adjacent tissue. Duct ectasia may be secondary to occlusion of duct lumina by hyperplastic lesions or intraductal neoplasms. Intraductal hyperplasia is the regular proliferation of

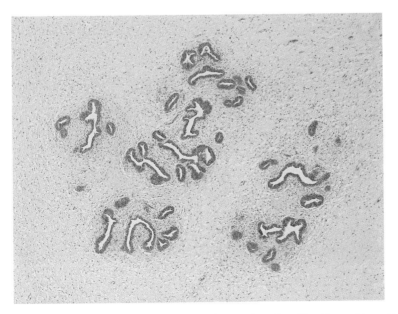

Figure 5.18   Feline mammary fibroadenomatous hyperplasia. The lesion consists of proliferative and branching mammary ducts lined by a simple columnar epithelium surrounded by an abundant, concentric proliferation of loose, edematous stroma.

epithelial cells within the lumen of ducts. The aggregates of cells may form small papillary projections or fill the duct lumina. The cells have hyperchromatic nuclei with little nuclear or cellular pleomorphism and scant cytoplasm. Larger lesions can be difficult to differentiate from in situ carcinoma.

Inflammatory Disease

Mastitis

Surgical pathology submission of mammary tissue with the primary complaint of mastitis is uncommon. However, inflammation may be observed in cases where mammary hyperplasia or neoplasia was suspected, or in tissue adjacent to mammary tumors or hyperplastic lesions. Mastitis as a primary disease typically occurs during the post-partum period or during pseudopregnancy. Mammary infection is usually ascending but occasionally develops following hematogenous spread. Initially, there is massive inter- and intra-alveolar infiltration of neutrophils, while the alveolar epithelium remains intact. Areas of healthy tissue may be interspaced with regions of intense inflammation. As the process continues, neutrophils may lyse and epithelial cells become degenerate leading to areas of complete alveolar destruction often with associated hemorrhage. As lesions become chronic, there is evidence of lymphocyte infiltration, alveolar destruction, and the early stages of fibrous tissue proliferation. Eventually, there will be extensive fibrosis with lymphocytic infiltration, shrunken or involuting alveoli, and thickened interlobular tissue.

Mammary Neoplasia

Mammary tumors have been described in virtually all mammalian species, including cetaceans. However, reports of spontaneous mammary tumors are uncommon in domestic species other than dogs, cats, and rats. In these species, there are considerable differences in mammary tumor incidence, type and biologic behavior. Mammary neoplasia may originate from epithelial cells lining ducts or alveoli, from myoepithelial cells, or from interstitial connective tissues, leading to a diverse array of mammary tumor types, which is particularly apparent in the dog.

Regardless of species, studies have demonstrated that hormones influence mammary tumor development, with OHE at a young age decreasing mammary tumor incidence, OHE at the time of tumor removal reducing the risk for developing subsequent mammary tumors in some species, and exposure to synthetic progestins in felines and zoo carnivores associated with an increased incidence of mammary tumors.

Rat Mammary Neoplasia

Mammary tissue in the rat is extensive and can be found ventrally, running from beneath the shoulder and chin area to the base of the tail, laterally on the neck, chest, and flanks, and dorsally on the neck and anterior chest. Tumors can arise anywhere that mammary tissue is present but most often occur on the abdomen and in the pit of the arm and groin. Females older than 18 months of age have a higher incidence of mammary tumors, and mammary tumors occasionally develop in male rats.

Mammary tumors are the most frequently occurring neoplasm in most strains of rats, where genetics appear to influence mammary tumor development. Rats most commonly develop benign mammary fibroadenomas (80–90%). In rats with malignant mammary tumors, local tissue invasion is slow to develop, and metastasis typically occurs late in the course of the disease.

Fibroadenoma

Fibroadenomas typically consist of lobules containing ductules, alveoli, or small cysts lined by a single layer of epithelium separated from other lobules by several layers of mature collagenous connective tissue. Epithelial cells generally have small nuclei, a single nucleolus, and often have cytoplasmic lipid vacuoles. These tumors have variable proportions of acinar and collagenous tissue. In some cases, the mass may consist primarily of connective tissue, with widely scattered acinar structures, while in other tumors, the epithelial component predominates. Focal areas of cellular pleomorphism may be present, and mast cells are frequently identified in the fibrous portion of the tumor. When complete excision is feasible, surgical removal is typically curative. However, in both females and males, tumors are likely to occur in other mammary glands (Figure 5.19).

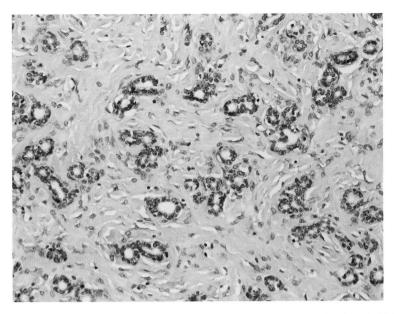

Figure 5.19 Rat mammary fibroadenoma. The tumor is composed of small ductules lined by simple cuboidal epithelium supported on an abundant collagenous connective tissue stroma.

Canine Mammary Neoplasia

Of our domestic species, canines are most frequently affected by mammary tumors. More than a quarter of unspayed female dogs will develop a mammary tumor during their lifetime. Disease is commonly multicentric, with the incidence of multiple tumors reported to be as high as 60%, and tumors in a single dog may be of more than one type. Many reports indicate that approximately half of the canine mammary tumors are malignant. However, the proportion of benign verses malignant tumors varies considerably between studies with 43.9–84% reported as benign verses 16–56.1% malignant To further complicate matters, when histologic malignancy is compared with behavioral malignancy in dogs, the ratio of histologically malignant cancers verses tumors with documented metastasis varied from 10 : 1 to 2 : 1.

Epidemiological and histopathological studies suggest that invasive mammary neoplasia in the dog is likely the end result of a histological continuum of progressive changes from benign to malignant resulting from hormonally driven carcinogenesis. The strong association between tumor size and malignancy, the low incidence of small malignant tumors, and the evidence of histological progression with increasing tumor size in dogs with multiple tumors all suggest that rather than developing as separate entities, malignant tumors most commonly arise from within benign neoplasms.

The most common mammary tumors in dogs are complex (tumors of epithelial and mesenchymal origin) or mixed tumors (tumors of epithelial and mesenchymal origin with differentiation toward cartilage and bone). There is considerable speculation as to the genesis of these complex mammary tumors. The observation that the epithelial and mesenchymal components of mixed mammary tumors are typically clonal supports the hypothesis that these two elements likely originate from stem cells with a high capacity for divergence.

Canine mammary neoplasia is one of the most challenging entities for the pathologist because of the complex histomorphology of mammary tumors, the existence of numerous distinct tumor types, expansion of the tumor within ducts, and the histologic continuum that exists beginning with hyperplastic lesions and progressing through malignant tumors. An in-depth discussion of the various types of canine mammary tumors is beyond the scope of this chapter and can be accessed in several reviews (see Goldschmidt et al.). Our understanding of the various factors that impact prognosis continues to evolve. In general, canine mammary tumors can be broadly divided into three categories: (i) benign, (ii) carcinomas within mixed tumors, and (iii) malignant mammary tumors.

Mammary Adenoma and Complex Mammary Adenoma (Mixed Tumor)

Benign mammary tumors: Benign mammary tumors are well-demarcated, and neoplastic cells do not extend beyond the basement membrane into the surrounding tissue. Cellularity is low to moderate, and anisokaryosis and anisocytosis are

(a)
(b)

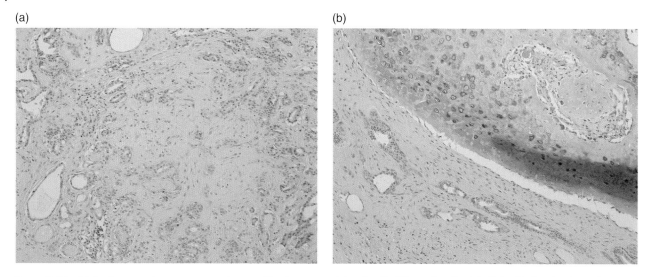

Figure 5.20   (a) Canine complex mammary adenoma. The tumor consists of well-differentiated epithelial cells forming irregular tubular structures accompanied by a sparse population of well-differentiated spindle cells supported on an abundant basophilic granular stroma. (b) Canine complex mammary adenoma. The tumor consists of well-differentiated epithelial cells forming irregular tubular structures accompanied by a sparse population of well-differentiated spindle cells supported on an abundant basophilic granular stroma admixed with islands of hyaline cartilage and bone.

minimal. Mitoses are rare, and there is the retention of cellular and nuclear polarity. Benign complex or mixed tumors are characterized by the presence of benign epithelial elements and mesenchymal cells forming myxoid fibrous tissue (complex), cartilage, and/or bone (mixed) (Figure 5.20a, b).

Malignant Mammary Neoplasia

Carcinoma within Mixed Tumors   Carcinomas within mixed tumors: Tumors with this designation account for 10–40% of the total number of diagnosed mammary carcinomas. The key morphological characteristic for the diagnosis of carcinoma within a mixed tumor is the presence of areas of invasion or microinvasion within a benign mixed tumor. The essential requirement to establish stromal invasion is the rupture of the basement membrane and the myoepithelial cell layer surrounding the carcinoma in situ. However, in some cases, the visualization of this area with standard stains is extremely difficult, and special stains, such as periodic acid Schiff (PAS) stains may aid in the identification of invasive foci in mixed mammary tumors of dogs. Because these tumors develop within an initially benign lesion, these neoplasms have a better prognosis and longer survival rates with an average survival time that is two to threefold higher than that of other canine mammary carcinomas.

Mammary Adenocarcinoma, Sarcoma, and Carcinosarcoma

Malignant mammary neoplasia can be derived from epithelial or mesenchymal tissue, or both. The most significant criteria for the diagnosis of malignant mammary tumors in the dog based on the gross assessment of the tumor and evaluation of H&E-stained sections includes tumor size, tumor type, significant nuclear and cellular pleomorphism, mitotic index, peritumoral tissue invasion, lymphovascular invasion, and regional lymph node (RLN) metastasis.

Tumor size has been found to be an independent prognostic factor in many different studies. Tumors smaller than 3 cm in diameter are associated with a significantly better prognosis than tumors larger than 3 cm. Tumors >5 cm in diameter are more likely to be malignant. Additionally, metastatic potential has been linked to tumor size. 86% of dogs with evidence of lymph node metastasis had tumors ≥5 cm in maximum diameter.

Complex carcinomas (composed of both epithelial and myoepithelial components) have a better prognosis than simple carcinomas, while sarcomas have the least favorable prognosis. In one study in which tumor type was compared to survival percentage, 40% of dogs with complex carcinomas, 18% of dogs with simple carcinomas, and 11% of dogs with sarcomas survived to the two-year post-surgical time point. In simple carcinomas, there is increasing malignancy from tubulopapillary to solid to anaplastic subtypes (Figure 5.21a–c).

Mitotic index, nuclear and cellular pleomorphism are generally incorporated into tumor grade. Criteria used to grade canine mammary tumors continues to evolve but generally includes the percentage of tubular formation, mitotic count,

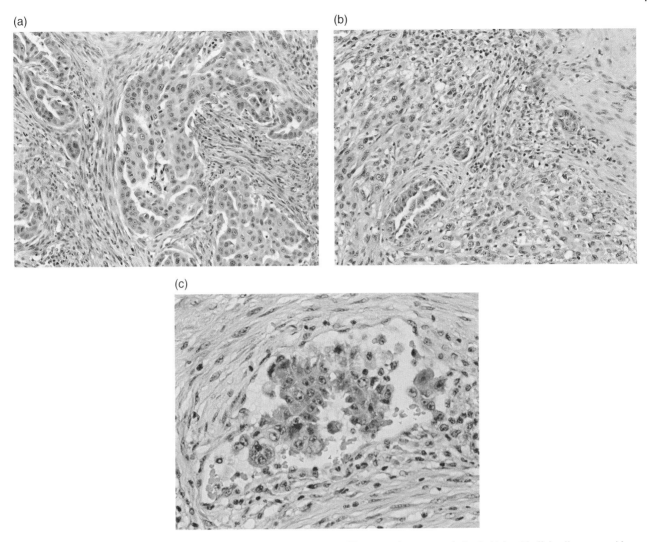

Figure 5.21 (a) Canine adenocarcinoma and malignant myoepithelioma. The tumor is composed of cuboidal epithelial cells arranged in solid clusters and irregular tubular structures accompanied by a moderately dense proliferation of spindle cells with large vesiculate nuclei, anisokaryosis, anisocytosis, and mitotic figures. (b) Canine mammary adenocarcinoma. The tumor is composed of an invasive population of epithelial cells arranged in irregular tubules and solid clusters supported on a fine fibrovascular stroma. (c) Canine mammary adenocarcinoma with lymphovascular invasion. Endothelium-lined vascular structures contain small clusters of neoplastic epithelial cells.

and nuclear morphology. In one study (Pena et al. 2012), the histological grade was significantly associated with several important prognostic indicators. With grade I tumors, only 3.4% recurred or metastasized, and none resulted in cancer mortality during the follow-up period (at least 28 months). For grade II tumors, 15.8% recurred or metastasized and resulted in cancer mortality during the follow-up period (at least 28 months). For grade III tumors, 58.8% recurred or metastasized and resulted in cancer mortality during the follow-up period (at least 28 months). Regarding disease-free survival (DFS), grade I tumors had a mean of 37.29 months, grade II tumors of 32.68 months, and grade III tumors of 7.78 months. Histological grade was significantly associated ($P < 0.001$) with the development of recurrences and/or metastases as 71.42% of the neoplasms that recurred or metastasized were grade III.

In canine mammary carcinomas, the degree of infiltration has been found to be of prognostic significance. When invasive tumors were compared with tumors exhibiting expansive growth, 8.3% of tumors with expansive growth recurred or metastasized, whereas 39.3% of tumors with invasive growth recurred or metastasized. The mean overall survival (OS) for dogs with expansive tumors was 23.3 months and only 8.3% died or were euthanized due to mammary neoplasia, whereas in dogs with invasive tumors, the OS was 19.3 months and 32.8% of dogs died or were euthanized due to mammary neoplasia.

Canine mammary carcinomas usually metastasize through the lymphatic system to the RLNs and subsequently to the lung or, less frequently, other organs (liver, kidneys, spleen, and bone). RLN metastases were significantly associated with shorter OS and DFS times, increased risk of recurrence/distant metastasis, and tumor-related death. 21.3% of dogs without RLN metastasis had local recurrence or distant metastases, whereas 47.4% of dogs with evidence of RLN metastasis had local recurrence or distant metastases.

The presence or absence of lymphovascular invasion is prognostically significant. In one study, dogs with lymphatic invasion had a shorter MST = 5 months, 1-year survival rate = 19%, and 2-year survival rate = 0%, when compared with dogs without lymphatic invasion, MST not reached, 1-year survival rate = 84%, 2-year survival rate = 69%. Dogs with lymphovascular invasion more frequently developed distant metastases (88 vs 25%) and local recurrence (31 vs 13%).

Feline Mammary Neoplasia

Mammary tumors are common in cats, comprising approximately 17% of all feline neoplasms, but mammary tumor prevalence in cats is 7.8 times less than in dogs. The mean age for the development of feline mammary tumors is between 10 and 12 years, with increasing risk up to 14 years of age. While queens are most commonly affected, mammary tumors have also been described in male cats, where their aggressive behavior is similar to mammary tumors in females.

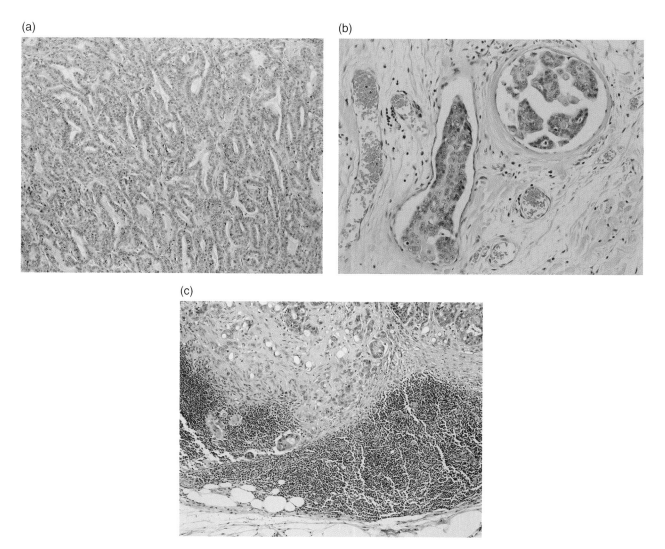

Figure 5.22 (a) Feline mammary adenocarcinoma. The tumor consists of an invasive proliferation of low columnar epithelial cells forming irregular tubular structures supported on a fine, fibrovascular stroma. (b) Feline mammary adenocarcinoma with lymphovascular invasion. Endothelium-lined vascular structures contain small clusters of neoplastic epithelial cells. (c) Lymph node metastasis from a feline mammary adenocarcinoma. A RLN is extensively effaced and replaced by a population of epithelial cells arranged in irregular tubules and solid clusters supported on a moderate fibrovascular stroma.

Feline Mammary Carcinoma/Adenocarcinoma

Malignant feline mammary tumors typically have aggressive biological behavior and a poor prognosis attributable to high rates of local recurrence and metastasis. When compared with canine mammary tumors, feline mammary tumors are much less heterogeneous and are typically simple neoplasms composed of only one cell type. Reports indicate that 80–96% of mammary tumors in cats are malignant, with metastatic rates ranging from 50 to 90%. RLNs (83%), lungs (83%), liver (25%), and pleura (22%) are the most commonly reported metastatic sites.

Although feline mammary carcinomas tend to be biologically aggressive, survival time in affected cats is variable with several parameters influencing survival time. For the pathologist, lymph node involvement, lymphovascular invasion, tumor size, and tumor grade have been demonstrated to be important prognostic indicators. Cats with demonstrable lymph node involvement had a median survival time of 5 months compared to 13 months for cats lacking evidence of lymph node metastasis. There is a strong correlation between lymphovascular invasion/emboli and OS. Cats without evidence of lymphovascular invasion/emboli had an OS of 28.8–36 months compared to an OS of 6.5–7 months for animals with demonstrable lymphovascular invasion/emboli. Prognosis has also been shown to be influenced by tumor size, as measured by tumor diameter or volume. A cutoff of 3-cm tumor diameter was found to be prognostically significant for OS. Cats with larger tumors (>3 cm) had a mean OS of five months compared to nine months for cats with smaller tumors. Lastly, there is a significant association between tumor grade and DFS. Grade 1 tumors had a DFS of 31 months, grade 2 DFS of 18 months, and grade 3 tumors with a DFS of 4 months. Tumor-related death rates after the first post-surgical year were 0% in cats with grade 1 tumors, 42.4% in those with grade 2 tumors, and (100%) in those with grade 3 tumors (Figure 5.22a–c).

References and Additional Readings

Bertagnolli, A.C., Soares, P., van Asch, B. et al. (2009). An assessment of the clonality of the components of canine mixed mammary tumours by mitochondrial DNA analysis. *Vet. J.* 182 (2): 269–274.

Canadas, A., França, M., Pereira, C. et al. (2019). Canine mammary tumors: comparison of classification and grading methods in a survival study. *Vet. Pathol.* 56 (2): 208–219.

Castagnaro, M., Casalone, C., Bozzetta, E. et al. (1998). Tumour grading and the one-year post-surgical prognosis in feline mammary carcinomas. *J. Comp. Pathol.* 119 (3): 263–275.

Chang, S.C., Chang, C.C., Chang, T.J. et al. (2005). Prognostic factors associated with survival two years after surgery in dogs with malignant mammary tumors: 79 cases (1998–2002). *J. Am. Vet. Med. Assoc.* 227 (10): 1625–1629.

Chocteau, F., Mordelet, V., Dagher, E. et al. (2021). One-year conditional survival of dogs and cats with invasive mammary carcinomas: a concept inspired from human breast cancer. *Vet. Comp. Oncol.* 19 (1): 140–151.

Christensen, B.W., Schlafer, D.H., Agnew, D.W. et al. (2012). Diagnostic value of transcervical endometrial biopsies in domestic dogs compared with full-thickness uterine sections. *Reprod. Domest. Anim.* 47 (Suppl 6): 342–346.

Dagher, E., Abadie, J., Loussouarn, D. et al. (2019). Feline invasive mammary carcinomas: prognostic value of histological grading. *Vet. Pathol.* 56 (5): 660–670.

Garcia-Iglesias, M.J., Am, B.-M., Perez-Martinez, C. et al. (1995). Incidence and pathomorphology of uterine tumours in the cow. *Zentralbl. Veterinarmed. A* 42 (7): 421–429.

Gelberg, H.B. and McEntee, K. (1984). Hyperplastic endometrial polyps in the dog and cat. *Vet. Pathol.* 21 (6): 570–573.

Goldschmidt, M., Peña, L., Rasotto, R. et al. (2011). Classification and grading of canine mammary tumors. *Vet. Pathol.* 48 (1): 117–131.

Kita, C., Chambers, J.K., Tanabe, M. et al. (2022). Immunohistochemical features of canine ovarian papillary adenocarcinoma and utility of cell block technique for detecting neoplastic cells in body cavity effusions. *J. Vet. Med. Sci.* 84 (3): 406–413.

Knauf, Y., Köhler, K., Knauf, S. et al. (2018). Histological classification of canine ovarian cyst types with reference to medical history. *J. Vet. Sci.* 19 (6): 725–734.

Mathieu, A. and Garner, M.M. (2021). A retrospective study of neoplasia in nondomestic felids in human care, with a comparative literature review. *J. Zoo. Wildl. Med.* 52 (2): 413–426.

Mayayo, S.L., Bo, S., and Pisu, M.C. (2018). Mammary fibroadenomatous hyperplasia in a male cat. *JFMS Open Rep.* 4 (1): 2055116918760155.

McIntyre, R.L., Levy, J.K., Roberts, J.F. et al. (2010). Developmental uterine anomalies in cats and dogs undergoing elective ovariohysterectomy. *J. Am. Vet. Med. Assoc.* 237 (5): 542–546.

Meyers-Wallen, V.N. (2012). Gonadal and sex differentiation abnormalities of dogs and cats. *Sex Dev.* 6 (1–3): 46–60.

Miller, M.A., Kottler, S.J., Cohn, L.A. et al. (2001). Mammary duct ectasia in dogs: 51 cases (1992–1999). *J. Am. Vet. Med. Assoc.* 218 (8): 1303–1307.

Mills, S.W., Musil, K.M., Davies, J.L. et al. (2015). Prognostic value of histologic grading for feline mammary carcinoma: a retrospective survival analysis. *Vet. Pathol.* 52 (2): 238–249.

Misdorp, W., Romijn, A., and Hart, A.A. (1991). Feline mammary tumors: a case-control study of hormonal factors. *Anticancer Res.* 11 (5): 1793–1797.

Morris, J. (2013). Mammary tumours in the cat: size matters, so early intervention saves lives. *J. Feline Med. Surg.* 15 (5): 391–400.

Noroozzadeh, M., Behboudi-Gandevani, S., Mosaffa, N. et al. (2019). High prevalence of benign mammary tumors in a rat model of polycystic ovary syndrome during postmenopausal period. *Gynecol. Endocrinol.* 35 (8): 679–684.

Orfanou, D.C., Ververidis, H.N., Pourlis, A. et al. (2009). Post-partum involution of the canine uterus – gross anatomical and histological features. *Reprod. Domest. Anim.* 44 (Suppl 2): 152–155.

Patnaik, A.K. and Greenlee, P.G. (1987). Canine ovarian neoplasms: a clinicopathologic study of 71 cases, including histology of 12 granulosa cell tumors. *Vet. Pathol.* 24 (6): 509–514.

Peña, L., De Andrés, P.J., Clemente, M. et al. (2012). Prognostic value of histological grading in noninflammatory canine mammary carcinomas in a prospective study with two-year follow-up: relationship with clinical and histological characteristics. *Vet. Pathol.* 50 (1): 94–105.

Rasotto, R., Zappulli, V., Castagnaro, M. et al. (2012). A retrospective study of those histopathologic parameters predictive of invasion of the lymphatic system by canine mammary carcinomas. *Vet. Pathol.* 49 (2): 330–340.

Rasotto, R., Berlato, D., Goldschmidt, M.H. et al. (2017). Prognostic significance of canine mammary tumor histologic subtypes: an observational cohort study of 229 cases. *Vet. Pathol.* 54 (4): 571–578.

Renaudin, C.D., Kelleman, A.A., Keel, K. et al. (2021). Equine granulosa cell tumours among other ovarian conditions: diagnostic challenges. *Equine Vet. J.* 53 (1): 60–70.

Rota, A., Ballarin, C., Vigier, B. et al. (2002). Age dependent changes in plasma anti-Mullerian hormone concentrations in the bovine male, female, and freemartin from birth to puberty: relationship between testosterone production and influence on sex differentiation. *Gen. Comp. Endocrinol.* 129 (1): 39–44.

Santos, A.A., Lopes, C.C., Ribeiro, J.R. et al. (2013). Identification of prognostic factors in canine mammary malignant tumours: a multivariable survival study. *BMC Vet. Res.* 4 (9): 1.

Sarli, G., Preziosi, R., Benazzi, C. et al. (2002). Prognostic value of histologic stage and proliferative activity in canine malignant mammary tumors. *J. Vet. Diagn. Investig.* 14: 25–34.

Sasidharan, J.K., Patra, M.K., Singh, L.K. et al. Ovarian cysts in the bitch: an update. *Top Companion Anim. Med.* 43: 100511.

Schlafer, D.H. (2012). Diseases of the canine uterus. *Reprod. Domest. Anim.* 47 (Suppl 6): 318–322.

Schlafer, D.H. and Gifford, A.T. (2008). Cystic endometrial hyperplasia, pseudo-placentational endometrial hyperplasia, and other cystic conditions of the canine and feline uterus. *Theriogenology* 70 (3): 349–358.

Schulman, F.Y., Goldschmidt, M.H., Hardcastle, M. et al. (2022). Teat sinus and duct adenomatous hyperplasia in dogs. *Vet. Pathol.* 59 (2): 256–263.

Snider, T.A., Sepoy, C., and Holyoak, G.R. (2011). Equine endometrial biopsy reviewed: observation, interpretation, and application of histopathologic data. *Theriogenology* 75 (9): 1567–1581.

Sontas, H.B., Stelletta, C., Milani, C. et al. (2011). Full recovery of subinvolution of placental sites in an American Staffordshire terrier bitch. *J. Small Anim. Pract.* 52 (1): 42–45.

Sorenmo, K.U., Kristiansen, V.M., Cofone, M.A. et al. (2009). Canine mammary gland tumours; a histological continuum from benign to malignant; clinical and histopathological evidence. *Vet. Comp. Oncol.* 7 (3): 162–172.

Stone, E.A. (1985). Urogenital tumors. *Vet. Clin. North Am. Small Anim. Pract.* 15 (3): 597–608.

Sorenmo, K.U., Kristiansen, V.M., Cofone, M.A. et al. (2009). Canine mammary gland tumours; a histological continuum from benign to malignant; clinical and histopathological evidence. *Vet. Comp. Oncol.* 7 (3): 162–172.

Vanholder, T., Opsomer, G., and de Kruif, A. (2006). Aetiology and pathogenesis of cystic ovarian follicles in dairy cattle: a review. *Reprod. Nutr. Dev.* 46 (2): 105–119.

Woodhouse, S.J. and Hanley, C.S. (2011). What is your diagnosis? Uterine adenocarcinoma. *J. Am. Vet. Med. Assoc.* 238 (3): 289–290.

Zappulli, V., Rasotto, R., Caliari, D. et al. (2015). Prognostic evaluation of feline mammary carcinomas: a review of the literature. *Vet. Pathol.* 52 (1): 46–60.

Index